# A Pocket Tour™ of Health & Fitness on the Internet

Jeanne C. Ryer

San Francisco • Paris • Düsseldorf • Soest

SYBEX

| | |
|---:|:---|
| *Pocket Tour Concept:* | Brenda Kienan |
| *Acquisitions Manager:* | Kristine Plachy |
| *Developmental Editor:* | Brenda Kienan |
| *Editor:* | Pat Coleman |
| *Project Editor:* | Malcolm Faulds |
| *Technical Editor:* | Jack Blacketter |
| *Book Designer:* | Emil Yanos |
| *Desktop Publisher:* | Dina F Quan |
| *Production Assistant:* | Taris Duffié |
| *Indexer:* | Ted Laux |
| *Cover Designer:* | Joanna Kim Gladden |
| *Cover Illustrator:* | Mike Miller |

*For Phil, Emily, and Anne*

# Acknowledgments

No book is ever the work of a single individual, and this one is no exception, with many sets of hands (and able minds) helping it along the way.

First, I want to acknowledge my debt to a group of people I've never seen and have known only over the Internet and through their work on the Internet. Lee Hancock and Gary Malet of Health Matrix and the Medical List, Scott Yanoff of Scott Yanoff's Internet Connections, David Filo and Jerry Yang of Yahoo, and too many others to name have helped to catalog the Internet's explosion of health resources so that the rest of us could find them.

I want to thank my long-time friend and agent Gareth Eserksy for her encouragement, support, and occasional prodding. And I want to thank my friends at MV Communications who keep my Internet connection going and growing.

At Sybex, Brenda Kienan led the way with a great idea and helped focus the vision. Malcolm Faulds kept me on track, and Pat Coleman was the quintessential helpful copy editor. Dan Tauber and Jack Blacketter gave the manuscript a technical vetting. And in Production, Dina Quan and Taris Duffié did wonderful work in all too little time.

The greatest thanks, though, go to my husband Phil for making it possible for me to travel the Internet and write late into the night. Without his help and forbearance, not one word would ever get written. I thank too my daughter Emily, who entertained herself admirably, and usually patiently, while Mommy was busy on the computer. And finally, a special thanks to my sister Jackie.

# Table of Contents

# Introduction

Ever since my first days on the Internet, I've been amazed by the power and breadth of this network of networks—a strand of thoughts, documents, and voices with no visible beginning or end. But even an apparently limitless resource can be limiting if its resources are uncharted, its documents uncatalogued, and its voices blended into a cacophonous muddle.

No matter how many years one has logged on the Internet, it's still a challenge to find the information you need when you need it. Some of the Internet's true pioneers have helped chart and catalog resources for the rest of us. Their task has become ever more daunting as both the resources and the number of users grow exponentially. It's been a pleasure and an honor, really, to follow along and make another contribution.

As the wealth of health and fitness information on the Internet has grown, so too has the need to help people find what's there and understand how to use it. There is probably no better use for the Internet, and no use better suited to the medium, than assembling and communicating information to people about their health and well-being.

The explosion of health and fitness resources on the Net bears that out. New resources are appearing every day. Major medical centers have discovered the usefulness of the Internet in organizing and communicating medical information to students, to patients, and to health-care professionals. Resources such as Virtual Hospital and OncoLink have led the way in presenting solid health information to diverse audiences and pushing the medium a bit to do it.

The U.S. government has been in the forefront of electronic communication and has made significant strides in making the documents and resources of U.S. health agencies readily available online. Many federal agencies have had online bulletin boards for some time, but tying them to the Internet and adding Gopher and World Wide Web connectivity has made the resources more reachable and more usable. It's also made the government more accessible. The Food and Drug Administration, for example, makes all of its regulations and its telephone book available online. No longer do you have to wait through interminable voice mail or phone tag to get to the person or the information you need. The U.S. health agencies have always generated health information for a consumer audience, but much of it moldered away unread. The Internet has made that information infinitely more accessible to those of us who need it, and there's never a fee or a delay in getting it.

The Internet has its "mom-and-pop" resources too, for example, the terrific FAQs (Frequently Asked Questions)—documents that sum up the accumulated wisdom of newsgroup members on health and other topics. And new to the Internet are the commercial sites, the best of which offer something of interest along with something to sell.

The Internet is also at its best when it brings people together; and when it comes to health concerns, that facet of the Net really shines. Whether it's moral support in the struggle to stop smoking or control weight, or emotional support in the face of cancer or depression, the people of the Internet touch one another's lives with generosity and compassion. Many times, in the course of reviewing e-mail discussion lists and newsgroups for this book, I have been moved by the courage of those facing serious illness and by the way they reach out over the Internet to help one another, even when gravely ill themselves.

Sorting out all these great new resources for this book has been a big task, but one that's been a lot of fun as well. It has also been a balancing act to find thorough and accurate information that's been written in understandable language and presented well. I have tried to present a range of resources and viewpoints; not everyone in the health-care community will agree with the information presented in each of these resources, particularly with the information in the section on alternative health care. It is especially important to use the information presented in these resources in the context of care from your health-care provider. Use these resources as a supplement to your regular care, not as a substitute for it.

## CONVENTIONS USED IN THIS BOOK

Before you start, you should note that there are several text and formatting conventions used in this book to make it a more convenient and easy-to-use resource. In the text itself, program font denotes Internet site addresses. Sometimes site addresses will span more than one line because of the limits of the book's margins; when using site addresses, just ignore such line breaks and enter the addresses exactly as they appear in the book. Underlining indicates hypertext; these are links found within World Wide Web pages that, once clicked, connect you to other documents or Internet sites. In a few places, **boldface** sets off any commands that you should type at your keyboard.

Notes, Tips, and Warnings appear at various points in the text to help guide your tour of the Internet:

*Notes provide additional background and context on the present topic or a related one.*

*Tips help you navigate the Internet more efficiently.*

*Warnings point out possible hazards and alert you to precautions that you should take.*

In **Part Two**, the section devoted to specific Internet sites, special icons will help you distinguish the various types of resources available.

This icon directs you to access the site through the World Wide Web.

This icon directs you to access the site through Usenet.

This icon directs you to access the site through FTP.

This icon directs you to access the site through Gopher.

This icon directs you to access the site through Telnet.

This icon indicates that the resource is an e-mail list server.

## TO YOUR HEALTH

The Internet health and fitness resources are vast and growing, the presentations improve every day, and the tools to search and use the Internet are becoming easier and easier to use. So, with *A Pocket Tour* in hand, enjoy your journey around the health and fitness resources on the Internet.

# Part One:
# The Basics

1

# A Voyage of Discovery

Ahead of you is a long and pleasant voyage exploring the Internet's vast resources on health and fitness. Depending on your time and interests, your voyage can be a series of short hops and frequent ports of call or a long journey packed with interesting people and some adventures. And you're *bound* to have a few adventures along the way. Serendipity plays a big part in Internet travel: A resource here leads you to another there; one newsgroup posting points you to still another. And the Internet's legendary climate of sharing applies to helping others along the way. You'll find lots of people willing to steer you in the right direction, as long as you ask your questions in the right places.

Even though the Internet is a lot more "user friendly" than it used to be, you will still bounce over some potholes and run into occasional dead ends. The Internet has been likened to a library that has no card catalog or to a city that has no street signs or maps. Internet navigational tools, such as Gopher and the World Wide Web (WWW), have made travel a lot easier, but don't be surprised if you occasionally hit a few frustrating bumps in the road.

What you find will be worth the trip. The Internet's resources on health and fitness have been expanding by the day. Whether you're interested in healthy living, fitness, exercise, and nutrition or whether you need help coping with some of life's health challenges, you'll find information and support on the Internet. You can find information on everything from exercise and eating to smoking and sleeping (see Figure 1.1). There are great resources on everyday ailments and also support for the big, serious illnesses. Online support and self-help groups cover topics as wide ranging as menopause, diabetes, carpal tunnel syndrome, and dealing with grief.

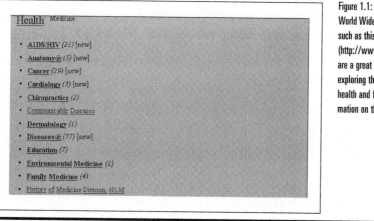

Figure 1.1:
World Wide Web sites,
such as this one at Yahoo
(http://www.yahoo.com),
are a great entry point for
exploring the wealth of
health and fitness infor-
mation on the Internet.

# EVALUATING WHAT YOU FIND

The health and fitness resources on the Internet vary in breadth, depth, clarity, and accuracy. How do you evaluate the quality of the information?

**Consider the source.** Information from a well-known medical school's Gopher or WWW pages is probably reliable.

**Find out if it has been published.** Where? Health professionals rely heavily on a process called *peer review* to screen articles before they're published in medical journals. There are even some peer-reviewed journals now published online.

Determine how old the information is. Some health fields change more rapidly than others. Descriptions of causes and symptoms usually change less rapidly than treatments.

**Use your common sense.** If a health claim sounds too good to be true, it probably is.

**Use the Net to verify information.** A quick posting to the relevant mailing list or newsgroup should get you some helpful feedback.

*Information from the Internet should never take the place of medical care or advice from your own physician. Use Internet resources to add to your knowledge, to broaden your understanding, and to get support from others in similar circumstances. And beware of the occasional charlatan. The recent influx of commercial activity on the Net has brought with it the online equivalent of snake-oil hucksters who may offer you advice and then try to sell you their magic potion. Many competent, ethical health professionals on the Net will be happy to point you toward helpful resources. None of them will ever attempt an online diagnosis or suggest treatment for a person they've never seen!*

## WHAT IS THE INTERNET?

The Internet is an international network of networks spanning all seven continents and well over a hundred countries; it is a confederation of thousands of networks connecting millions of computers. Sometimes it's easier to describe what the Internet *is not* than what it *is*. The Internet is *not* just one network. It is *not* owned or funded by any one institution, organization, or government. It is *not* a commercial service.

> *Sometimes it's easier to describe what the Internet is not than what it is.*

The Internet is a voluntary network for which the participants agree to use common protocols and a common set of ground rules so that, working together, everything runs smoothly. It's unlikely you would ever find a piece of hardware stamped "Property of the Internet," because the Internet does not exist as an entity or organization.

The Internet got its start as a research network linking the military with government contractors, many of whom were at large universities. What began as a project to share computer resources across institutions soon mushroomed as more people at these institutions discovered the enormous utility of a network that linked them with colleagues across the country and then around the world.

Access to the Internet for individuals is a fairly recent phenomenon, but then everything to do with the Internet is really a recent phenomenon. The Internet has grown at exponential rates (see Figure 1.2) and changed in ways that its original designers might never have predicted. What was once an online haven for computer jocks, researchers, and academics is now open to the rest of us.

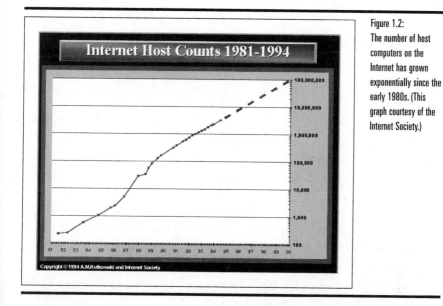

Figure 1.2:
The number of host computers on the Internet has grown exponentially since the early 1980s. (This graph courtesy of the Internet Society.)

*The Internet is like a city under constant construction. Resources may be here today and somewhere else tomorrow. All resources in this book were up to date as of press time, but by the time you read this, their addresses or locations may have changed, and in a few cases, resources may have even ceased to exist.*

In the Internet's long-standing tradition of sharing, new documents, resources, and tools are being made available all the time. The depth and breadth of the resources on the Internet have grown almost as quickly as the number of users. Whatever your interest, you can probably find information about it and other people who share your passion somewhere on the Internet.

# Getting to the Internet

Until recently, Internet access wasn't always easy unless you worked for a major university or a big government contractor. Some public access providers served bigger cities and high-tech centers, but most of the rest of the country was left without an on-ramp to the proverbial information highway.

Now, if you can get to a phone line, you can access the Internet. Although the level of access and its costs may vary tremendously, no one in this country within reach of a telephone line (or a cellular link) needs to live without the wealth of Internet resources.

## WHAT DO YOU NEED?

In addition to that telephone line, you need at least a basic computer, a modem, and a communications software package. The faster and newer your computer and modem, the better, but plenty of people access the Internet regularly from computers that would bring $25 at a yard sale.

If you're lucky enough to work where Internet access is provided on your office workstation, you won't have to worry too much about which hardware and software configurations will get you the most for your access dollar. If you're on your own, generally speaking, the fastest, newest modem you can get should be your choice for Internet use, but don't spend money for a modem faster than one your computer will support. If you find you must pay for access time and telephone charges by the minute, and you plan to be online a lot and download big files, investing in a faster modem will probably be worth it. If, however, you're only a local call from your Internet access provider and your budget is tight, a less-than-state-of the-art modem will do for most Internet applications.

The big exception to all the above—and on the Internet, there's always an exception that proves the rule—is WWW access. World Wide Web is the latest and greatest in Internet applications. Although it's possible to access WWW in a text form with a slow modem, WWW requires, to be its graphical best, a direct Internet connection (more on that in a minute) and a minimum of a 14,400 bps modem (and preferably faster). WWW browser software needs a minimum of a 386 or equivalent computer, and, of course, a 486 would be better.

*Many online services currently support only 9,600 or 14,400 bps access. In that case, your slick new 28,800 bps modem has to step down its speed to match that of the providers. All the services are upgrading their access speeds, but don't assume your service provider will necessarily be able to match your modem speed.*

The software you need depends a bit on your level and type of Internet access. For basic dial-up Internet access, you can get by with the kind of simple communications software package that usually comes bundled with your modem. Of course, the more features the better; you can waste a lot of expensive online time if your software doesn't support your modem's highest speed or the better file transfer protocols.

The next level of software includes offline electronic mail-reader programs. Some of these have been available online as *shareware*, software made available by its authors in the expectation you'll pay for it if you use it, and recently have come to the commercial market. Assuming your Internet access provider will support one, offline readers are invaluable time and money savers. Some commercial online services provide offline mail and news programs. Whatever their features, they certainly beat trying to manage your mail during valuable online time.

A number of Internet software suites have recently come to the market; most are preconfigured for some of the larger Internet access providers. They generally offer a package of Internet tools and *client* programs that allow you to use e-mail, file transfer, news, Gopher, Telnet, and more. Most now offer a WWW browser as well (see Figure 1.3). Before you buy, you'll want to look at the software tools and their ease of use, the network access that providers support, whether those providers are economical for your location and kind of use, and how easily the products can be configured to your existing provider or special situation.

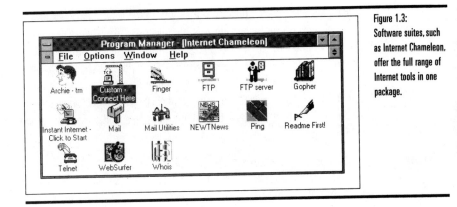

Figure 1.3:
Software suites, such as Internet Chameleon, offer the full range of Internet tools in one package.

# HOW TO GET THERE

Right now you can get to the Internet in four ways: direct access, SLIP/PPP access, dial-up accounts, and commercial online services. What you can do on the Internet—how far you can travel, how easily, and how much it will cost—depends greatly on the type of access. If you live in a major metropolitan area, you'll probably have choices. You can use your good-consumer skills to weigh options for services, costs, and ease of use. If you live in a small town or in a rural area, your decision will probably be driven by the cost of the phone connection to get to 'the system that gets you to the Internet. Look for providers with local access numbers first. If you can't find one, explore some of the pay-as-you-go 800 services, calling plans from your local or long distance phone company, or services such as Sprint's PC Pursuit or the CompuServe Packet Network.

*To learn more about the Internet, see Appendix A for a list of Internet resources and references.*

*To get onto the Internet, see Appendix B for a list of major Internet service providers.*

# DIRECT ACCESS

Easiest of all is direct access to the Internet from a network where you work. Once the province of large universities and government contractors, Internet access is now considered a necessity by many companies, large and small.

Your company-provided access may come as full-fledged, full-time access to the Internet with a complete set of client programs that make it easy for you to use all the Internet's resources. If you work in a smaller company, your access may be limited, perhaps only electronic mail. Because your employer is probably paying a flat rate (although a big one) for the Internet connection, it's not likely that your personal use will be monitored, unless, of course, you play too many interactive games on company time! Some companies and government offices, however, do strictly limit Internet access to work-related activities, so be sure you understand the policy where you work.

## SLIP AND PPP ACCOUNTS

Even if you're on your own, you can have direct Internet access through what's called a SLIP or PPP account with an Internet service provider. SLIP, which stands for Serial Line Interface Protocol, and PPP, which stands for Point-to-Point Protocol, are essentially dial-up direct access to the Internet allowing you to use a full suite of client programs, such as software to browse the World Wide Web, over a regular telephone line. The software you need is available in commercial packages (see Figure 1.4) or as shareware you can download from the Internet. Be aware that configuring shareware to work with both your system and your Internet access provider's system will take some time and some understanding of Internet networking vocabulary and concepts. If you're a novice, spending a hundred dollars or so for commercial software could save you hours and hours of frustration. Even configuring some commercial packages can take patience; so don't try it the night before a big project deadline.

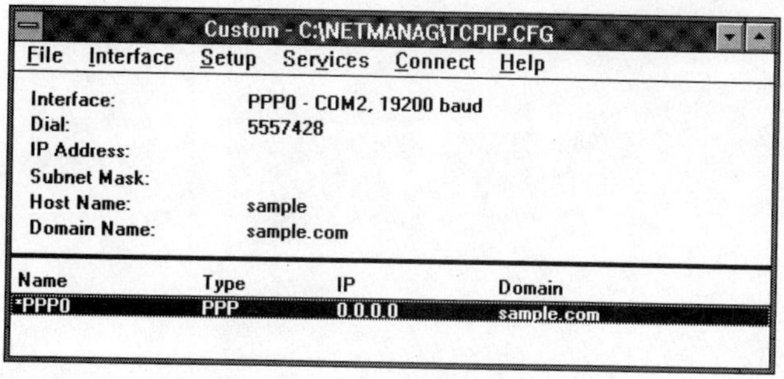

Figure 1.4:
Internet access software such as Internet Chameleon can help you configure your own direct access SLIP or PPP account.

You will need to locate an Internet service provider within an economical calling area and then configure your system to its requirements. As we mentioned earlier, several software developers and commercial Internet service providers have recently begun teaming up to provide preconfigured SLIP/PPP access that will work right out of the box.

## DIAL-UP ACCOUNTS

Many Internet access companies offer *dial-up,* or *shell,* accounts on the Internet. With a dial-up account, you use your regular telephone line to access the Internet through the company's network connection. Dial-up accounts come in two basic flavors—plain vanilla and fancy.

The plain vanilla version usually gives you modem access to a Unix-based system, an account number, and a password. That system generally has a full range of Internet tools, such as e-mail, news, Telnet, and Gopher. Dial-up accounts generally don't support a graphical WWW, although they may provide some alternatives. They are generally text-based systems. Most offer Gopher-like menus (see Figure 1.5); others simply present you with a Unix system prompt, and you have to know what to do next.

These systems have been known in Internet circles as public access Unix providers. Most public access Unix providers serve a specific local or regional area; a few have national 800 service or a network of local numbers.

 *A list of public access Unix providers, called PDIAL (Public Dialup Internet Access List), is updated periodically by Peter Kaminski. To get the list, send e-mail with the phrase Send PDIAL in the body of the message to info-deliserver@pdial.com.*

```
┌─────────────────────────────────────────────────────────┐
│         Internet Gopher Information Client v1.1█         │
│                                                          │
│            Root gopher server: gopher.mv.com             │
│    -> 1. Information and Getting Started <Hit RETURN here>/│
│       2. Utilities <Mail, News, etc.>/                   │
│       3. Internet Services to Explore/                   │
│       4. Games/                                          │
│       5. UNIX shell/                                     │
│       6. Suggestion Box, and Problem Reports/            │
│                                                          │
│                                                          │
│                                                          │
│ Press █ for Help, █ to Quit, █ to go up a menu   Page: 1 │
└─────────────────────────────────────────────────────────┘
```

Figure 1.5:
Most dial-up Internet service providers offer a Gopher menu or some other menu system to guide you to their services.

The fancy form of dial-up access is offered by companies, such as Netcom, PSI, and InterCon Systems, that have both proprietary client software and a network of local access numbers in major cities or an 800 number service. For your sign-up fee and monthly charges you usually get the software necessary for e-mail, news, Telnet, and so on and a defined number of online hours.

## COMMERCIAL ONLINE SERVICES

The major commercial online services, such as America Online, CompuServe, and Prodigy, are adding to their Internet services almost daily (see Figure 1.6). Only a few years ago, sending electronic mail messages to subscribers on the commercial networks was difficult and sometimes impossible. Now the three biggest services are joining Delphi, which has long had an Internet connection, in giving their subscribers access to the wealth of Internet resources. Services are being added and rates are changing too quickly to include them in this book. If you're shopping for access and think one of the commercial online services is right for you, look at which Internet services it has available now (as opposed to which are on the drawing board), check on surcharges for Internet services or e-mail, and find out about the ease of access in your telephone calling area.

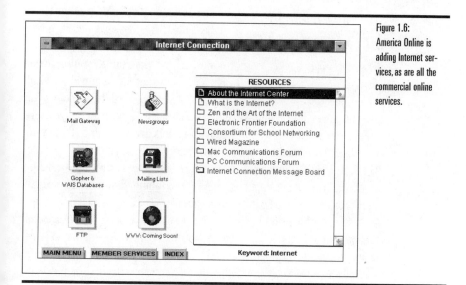

Figure 1.6: America Online is adding Internet services, as are all the commercial online services.

# What It Costs

Because it's a voluntary network, the Internet itself, once you're on it, doesn't really charge you anything at all. What you do pay for though, since there is no free lunch, is *access* to the Internet and, in some cases, the cost of a telephone connection to your access provider.

Costs of Internet access vary widely—and wildly. Depending on where you are and which access path you can choose, your costs can range from $5 a month to $10,000 and more a year. It's a little like comparing the cost of a bus token to a round-the-world cruise on the *QEII*. It all depends on where you are, where you're going, and how well you like to travel.

> *Depending on where you are and which access path you can choose, your costs can range from $5 a month to $10,000 and more a year.*

The first thing to evaluate—as we've hinted more than once—is the cost of the phone access to get to a provider or to set up as a direct Internet site yourself. If you have a local phone number access with unlimited message units, you're home free. If you're outside a provider's local calling area, you need to explore your long-distance calling options and find the cheapest. If you want the *QEII* version of Internet access, you'll need a dedicated data line—price those with your local phone company. Data lines vary widely in cost and capability. They can be pricey, and what you want may not always be readily available.

In terms of service options, as a rule of thumb, dial-up public access Unix providers tend to be the most economical. The commercial online services are probably next highest in price, depending a lot on your usage and their system of charges. Some charge for sending Internet e-mail, and some charge for receiving Internet e-mail. Your costs can add up quickly if you subscribe to a few Internet mailing lists. The commercial dial-up providers come in a little higher than that. Depending on your provider, SLIP and PPP access can run a close race with the commercial dial-up providers, but again, fee schedules vary, and your usage patterns will impact your costs as well. If you want a full direct Internet connection, you will have to pay handsomely for one of the regional networks to connect you, and you'll need the expertise to maintain the software and hardware to keep your connection running smoothly.

# Internet Lingo

Venturing into the Internet sometimes seems like an Alice in Wonderland journey into a land where the language sounds familiar but where the words don't mean quite the same things. If you begin to feel that the Internet is populated by a bunch of people with a fairly strange and punny sense of humor, well, you're probably right.

Internet-speak falls into a few main categories: alphabet-soup abbreviations and acronyms (FAQs, WAIS), plays on words (Gopher, archie), symbols (smileys and emoticons), resource addresses (URLs), and punctuation (the ubiquitous dot).

**Punctuation**   Let's start with the dot. All Internet addresses use a character that looks like a period (and types like one) to delineate the segments of the user name and the name of the domain (or where the computer is). It may look like a period, but it is a *dot* and is read out loud as "dot." For example, sybex.com is read out loud as *"sybex dot com."* The @ sign (pronounced "at") is every bit as important in addresses, and the slash (/) indicates directories and files.

Internet addresses are simple and straightforward. E-mail addresses give the addressee's username to the left of the @ sign and the name of the *domain* to the right; so it's username@computer.somewhere. Both sides of the address can have elements that are separated with dots. The *domain name* usually shows the name of the computer, or *host name*, and sometimes the name of the institution. The domain name always ends with the top-level domain, which usually indicates whether the domain is an educational institution (.edu), a business (.com), or another network (.net), to name a few. Top-level domains can also indicate the computer's home country, for example, .jp for Japan or .ch for Switzerland.

The form for addresses and locations of Internet resources used to be a bit inconsistent. The recent establishment of a standard *Uniform Resource*

*Locator (URL)* has improved things enormously. URLs consistently format resource addresses, showing the type of resource, the location, and the path to the directory (see Table 1.1). URLs have been used most widely to identify WWW resources. The more sophisticated client programs, such as WWW, Gopher, and FTP (File Transfer Protocol), have been able to take advantage of the URL format. If you use one of these client programs, all you need to do is type the URL; the program does all the work of getting you there. Even if you don't have a client program, the URL gives you all the information you need to access the resource.

| Table 1.1 Uniform Resource Locators (URLs) | |
|---|---|
| **Resource Type** | **Example** |
| World Wide Web | http://www.columbia.edu/cu/healthwise/ |
| Gopher | Gopher://riceinfo.rice.edu/Health and Safety at Rice/HealthInfo/ |
| File | ftp://vax8.cfsan.fda.gov |
| Telnet | telnet://fdabbs.fda.gov |

**Symbols**   The symbols, called *smileys* or *emoticons*, have an entire lexicon to themselves. Smileys originated to show emotion in a bland, text-based medium in which no voice inflection offers cues to the meaning of the message. In face-to-face conversation, people can usually tell when we're joking or being sarcastic by our facial expression and tone of voice. Not so in e-mail text, and more than a few have felt injured by what was intended to be witty repartee. The simplest symbol is the original smiley, spelled :-) and meant to connote a "just kidding" kind of grin. (If you don't get it, tip your head a little to the left and look again.) That simple symbol has evolved into a language of its own, with emoticons for every occasion, from winks to leers to pure indifference.

**Plays on Words**   The word-play terms come from a similar vein of humor. The originators of the Internet search tool archie (that lowercase *a* is correct) insist that the name was derived from the word *archive*. Since archie is a tool for finding things in FTP archives, its companion search program for Gopher, Veronica, must have been named for someone other than the comic strip character. And Jughead, another search tool, must not have any connection with either!

**Abbreviations and Acronyms** The Internet is awash with abbreviations and acronyms, from the serious to the not-so-serious. The most important to a newcomer is *FAQ*, short for Frequently Asked Questions. FAQs are documents compiled from common questions to newsgroups, mailing lists, or whatever. Other common abbreviations (although a list of them all would constitute a sizable dictionary) are *WWW* for World Wide Web and *WAIS* for Wide Area Information Server.

> *The Internet is awash with abbreviations and acronyms, from the serious to the not-so-serious.*

Some abbreviations substitute for common phrases used in newsgroup discourse. For example, IMHO means In My Humble Opinion; ROTFL means Rolling on the Floor Laughing. Most of these abbreviations originated in on-line chat as typing time-savers. Although keeping messages brief has merit, your readers may not understand all the abbreviations. Unless you're certain of your reader's level of alphabet-soup comprehension, it's probably fairer not to use abbreviations and acronyms.

# GLOSSARY

| | |
|---|---|
| *anonymous FTP* | Access to public file archives on the Internet. Derives from the sign-on procedure, which calls for the user id anonymous and your email address as a password. |
| *archie* | An Internet system of servers that searches for files in publicly available FTP archives. |
| *backbone* | The high-speed network connections of the Internet. |
| *bandwidth* | The size of the network "pipeline." |
| *BITnet* | An academic network and home to many e-mail discussion lists. Originally an acronym for the "Because It's Time Network." |
| *browser* | A program for accessing hypertext and hypermedia documents. |
| *client* | A program that accesses a computer for services or information. |
| *e-mail* | Electronic mail, or the process of sending and receiving messages over the Internet (or other network). |

| | |
|---|---|
| *emoticon* | A symbol or set of symbols used to convey emotion in text (*see* smiley). |
| *FAQ* | Frequently Asked Questions document; assembles answers to common questions for broad distribution. |
| *Finger* | A program to display user identification or other information. |
| *flame* | An angry interchange on the network. |
| *FTP* | File Transfer Protocol, the Internet tool for moving files from one location to another. Used to move files or documents from public systems to your own computer or account. |
| *FTPmail* | A version of FTP for electronic mail use. |
| *Gopher* | A menu-based tool for organizing and accessing network resources. |
| *Gopherspace* | The worldwide Gopher system. |
| *header* | The addressing information that directs your electronic mail message or newsgroup posting. |
| *home page* | A beginning point or central site on the World Wide Web. |
| *hypermedia* | Linked documents containing other media, for example, video and sound. |
| *hypertext* | Documents or data linked to other documents or data. |
| *Jughead* | A Gopher search program that searches a specific set of Gopher menus. |
| *link* | A connection between hypertext or hypermedia documents. |
| *Listproc* | A mailing list processing program. |
| *Listserv* | A mailing list management program. |
| *lurk* | The practice of reading a newsgroup or e-mail discussion list without joining in. |
| *Mailserv* | A mailing list processing prgram. |
| *mail server* | A computer that responds automatically to electronic mail requests for information documents, files, and so on. |
| *mailing list* | Group discussion via electronic mail. Mailing lists focus on specific topics of interest to the list members and are managed by Listservs or other mailing-list processing programs. |
| *Majordomo* | A mailing list processing program. |

| | |
|---|---|
| *nameserver* | A computer that manages user names, user identification, and Internet numeric addresses. |
| *netiquette* | The Internet code of conduct. |
| *newbie* | A new Internet user, often modified, as in "clueless newbie." |
| *newsgroup* | Electronic discussion groups. |
| *newsreader* | A program that presents and organizes Usenet news for the user. |
| *page* | A hypertext document on the World Wide Web. |
| *PPP* | Point-to Point Protocol, a protocol for direct Internet access over the telephone lines. |
| *protocol* | An agreement on or system for how computers will communicate, for example, File Transfer Protocol. |
| *server* | A computer that provides services on a network. |
| *shareware* | Software made available on the networks by the authors, who usually expect a modest payment from users after a trial period. |
| *shell* | A user interface program for accounts on Unix systems. |
| *signature (also .sig)* | A short file, usually appended to electronic mail messages, providing information about the sender. Often used for elaborate graphics, quotes, and personal statements. |
| *SLIP* | Serial Line Internet Protocol, a protocol for direct Internet access over a regular telephone line. |
| *smiley* | A typographic representation of emotion in text characters (*see* emoticon). |
| *spam* | (verb) To crosspost the same message (usually commercial) to numerous newsgroups. |
| *TCP/IP* | Transmission Control Protocol/Internet Protocol, the underlying protocols that define the Internet. |
| *Telnet* | A protocol to log in to remote computers on the Internet. Used to access databases, for example, or one's own accounts from a remote location. |
| *Unix* | A computer operating system common on the Internet. |
| *URL* | Uniform Resource Locator, a system of addressing Internet resources. |
| *Usenet* | The worldwide newsgroup network. |

| | |
|---|---|
| *Veronica* | A search program for Gophers. |
| *WAIS* | Wide Area Information Servers system for searching databases. |
| *Web* | The World Wide Web. |
| *Whois* | A program to search for user or network addresses. |
| *World Wide Web* | A program that connects network resources with hypertext links. |
| *WWW* | The World Wide Web. |

# The Local Customs

Even though it's young in years, the Internet has a well-defined culture. Unless you've been on the Net forever (in which case you probably wouldn't need this book), you're a relative Net newcomer, a stranger in a strange land. As a newcomer, you'd be wise to get the feel of the local customs before you get yourself in trouble. The Internet has a mostly unwritten code of conduct, called netiquette, that has evolved as a means of keeping a world without laws or police operating smoothly and peacefully. Don't get the idea, though, that "anything goes" on the Net. Beginners' stumbles are usually tolerated, but blatant violations will bring the wrath of your fellow netters down on your head and into your e-mail box.

Like most codes of conduct, netiquette is premised on treating others as one would like to be treated. Netiquette involves three basic principles: shared resources, conservation of resources, and civil behavior.

## SHARE AND SHARE ALIKE

Even though the Internet seems like a boundless resource, it is not. It runs on networks essentially owned by others; some of those networks are big, some aren't. And even the big ones have been stretched by enormous growth in use. So the principle of "conserve bandwidth" applies to all Net activity. That means you don't send a long message when a short one will do or send a huge software file that could have been compressed. It also means that you should use the resources closest to you. Don't use precious distant network resources when you could use those close to you. For example, don't tap an archie server in Japan when one in New Jersey is much closer to you.

> *The principle of "conserve bandwidth" applies to all Net activity.*

## SHOW RESPECT FOR THE RESOURCE

The second principle comes out of the shared resources ethos of the Net. Most resources available to you are there by the grace of the people who did the work and their sponsoring institutions. They don't owe you anything, as an outsider, but they're happy to share. Netiquette means doing your part by not using resources during peak times (it slows down their systems when they need them) or hogging resources by excessive use. More than a few neat resources have been taken off the Net because their use overtapped the sponsor's capabilities.

## MIND YOUR MANNERS

The Net's rules for civil behavior are based on common courtesy and respect for others. Some big no-nos include the following:

◆ Posting or forwarding private correspondence without the writer's consent.

◆ Sending junk mail, or "spamming," which means posting the same message to large numbers of newsgroups or mailing lists. Spamming commercial or business information is an especially big offense.

◆ Carrying on "flame wars" in public places. If you have an issue with someone, take care of it in private e-mail, not in the newsgroup or mailing list.

◆ Reposting chain letters or any of the "urban legends" that have been turning up on the Net for years. If you receive messages about Craig Shergold, the modem tax, the $250 cookie recipe, or Dave Rhodes, don't pass them on!

*Internet culture goes beyond good manners. The Internet has its heroes and its villains, its mythic characters, and its stories that refuse to die. If you want to know more about this new country you're visiting, check out some of the standard Internet references or sign on to mailing lists such as net-happenings (majordomo@ds.internic.net) or the newsgroups news.announce.newusers, alt.culture.internet, or alt.internet.services.*

# Internet Tools You Can Use

The Internet uses three standard tools: e-mail, FTP (file transfer protocol), and Telnet. Network navigators and search tools, such as Gopher, WWW, and WAIS, have been widely accepted and have been proliferating across the Net. Depending on your access, you may be able to use all or only some of these tools.

## ELECTRONIC MAIL

Electronic mail, or *e-mail,* is probably the Internet's most popular tool, and it is certainly a powerful communications medium. E-mail takes two basic forms: (1) the one-to-one interaction similar to regular, postal mail (see Figure 1.7); and (2) the one-to-many, many-to-one interaction of e-mail discussion lists.

Virtually every Internet access system has some kind of electronic mail program, called an *e-mail reade*r. Some are sophisticated and easy to use;

```
Received:  (8.6.10/mv(b)/mem-940616)
           id OAA26292 for <yourname@sample.com>; Thu, 30 Mar 1995 14:48:22 -
0500
Date: Thu, 30 Mar 95 11:59:06 PST
From:YourName@Sample.COM
Subject: Sample Message
X-Mailer: Chameleon - TCP/IP for Windows by NetManage, Inc.
Message-ID: <Chameleon.4.01.2.950330120233.r@>
MIME-Version: 1.0
Content-Type: TEXT/PLAIN; charset=US-ASCII

Hi.

I've been looking for health and fitness resources on the Internet.  Can
you help point me in the right direction?

Thanks!

----------------------------------------

E-mail: YourName@sample.com
Date:03/30/95
Time: 12:01:23
```

Figure 1.7:
A sample e-mail
message

a few aren't. They all, however, allow you to write a message, address it, send it, and receive a reply. Bells and whistles beyond that are common and include features such as address books, offline reading and writing of messages, folders in which to save and organize your incoming and outgoing mail, and nifty word-processing functions.

Once you have written and "mailed" your message, your Internet access provider's mail program packages your message for delivery through the system. Although e-mail is not instantaneous, it sometimes seems like it; often you'll get a response to a message you sent only moments ago. Some providers, however, batch mail and send it periodically throughout or at the end of the day. Be sure to check on your mail system. You won't want to wait around all day for an answer to a message that won't even go out until after 5 PM.

## E-MAIL BASICS

We can't begin to cover instructions for all e-mail readers in a book this size, and, really, e-mail is so easy to use that you can probably figure out the basics for yourself with your first message. Basically, you need four things:

◆ From: an address of your own, supplied usually with your account and inserted by your mail program,

◆ To: the address of your e-mail-ee,

◆ Re: or Subject: the topic, and

◆ Message: something to say.

 Use care in addressing e-mail messages! The most common cause of a bounced, or "returned as undeliverable," message is a simple typo in the address.

 Always use a brief but descriptive subject line in your e-mail. Many on the Internet receive tens or even hundreds of messages each day. A good subject line helps them sort their mail and prioritize their responses.

Many Net regulars add a .sig, or signature file, to all their messages, which gives some basic information about who and where they are, sometimes even

including favorite quotes and ASCII graphics. Some basic information is probably desirable, but .sig files should be kept to four lines or fewer.

On an incoming message, the *header* has some basic and valuable information:

◆ Date: the date and time the message was sent,

◆ From: the e-mail address, and sometimes the full name, of whoever sent it,

◆ Reply to: the list address, if the message came from a mailing list,

◆ To: your name and e-mail address or the names of the mailing list and its address,

◆ Subject: what it's about.

You'll probably find yourself using e-mail to communicate and request information from individuals, to join e-mail discussion lists, to correspond privately with people you meet on those lists, and to access other Internet resources.

## FINDING E-MAIL ADDRESSES

The simplest way to get a person's e-mail address is to call and ask! Lots of people have been working to generate Internet "phone books" of e-mail addresses, but the direct approach still works best. Failing that, and a check of the person's stationery or business card, a little educated guesswork is the next best tactic. You can try sending an "Are you there?" message with a standardized form of the person's name to the institution or company. Most large systems operate a name server that stores forms of individual names and directs e-mail to the proper account. For example, if you think your college friend Janie Doe is working at the big SRI think tank, you could try a message addressed to jane.doe@sri.com. Other approaches include using Finger, a program that displays user information from the user's home system, university directories of faculty and staff e-mail addresses in their Gopher servers, and Gopher servers with wide-ranging phone book sections in their menus. If you're still stumped, check some standard Internet references for instructions on whois, netfind, the X.500 official Internet "White Pages," and the knowbot system.

## E-MAIL DISCUSSION LISTS

In addition to the one-to-one communication, e-mail is an amazingly effective tool for groups of people to communicate with one another through e-mail discussion lists. E-mail discussion list programs come in a few varieties, depending on the software running on the system that hosts them. Called Listserv, Listproc, Mailserv, or Majordomo, these software programs have automated mailing list functions that allow folks of like interests to join in group discussions. Although the original Listserv program was developed for the BITnet network and not for the Internet at all, mailing list programs are often generically referred to as *listservs* or *listservers*. This is a little like calling tissues Kleenex, however, and that goes unappreciated by the programmers whose work is being genericized. Listserver programs handle the nitty-gritty functions of adding and deleting subscribers, routing mail, and so on. Some smaller Internet mailing lists are not automated, and a real person does some or all the tasks. Usually these lists have an administrative address that looks like mailinglistname-request@whereever.edu. No matter which system your chosen list uses, you get messages that are posted to the list by other members, and they get your messages.

> *When it comes to health and fitness information-sharing, these lists really shine.*

E-mail discussion lists are great for all kinds of professionals; they link colleagues together over continents. Hobbyists of all sorts love them because they provide a medium for unmatched information sharing. But when it comes to health and fitness information-sharing, these lists really shine. Where else could you find a ready-made group of people who care about what you care about, who share in your struggles, and who have helpful information that would be hard to find on your own?

So how do e-mail discussion lists work? Every list has a volunteer manager, called the *list owner,* who takes care of the business of the list and sets the general tone and topic of the discussion. List members can use the list to send their thoughts, opinions, and questions to all other list members, many of whom will, in turn, respond. Some lists are moderated, which means that a person, usually the list owner, reviews all messages for content and cogency before they make it to the list. Some lists are open to all comers; others limit membership to a particular group, usually professional, and have some sort of system for screening new subscribers.

Subscription business, such as subscribing, unsubscribing, and requesting a message *digest*—usually a day's worth of messages combined into one mailing—is sent to the administrative address. Messages to the mailing list members are sent to the list address. For example, the administrative address for FIT-L, a popular mailing list on health and fitness, is listserv@etsuadmn.etsu.edu. The address for posted messages to other members is fit-l@etsuadmn.etsu.edu. We've included the address and syntax for subscribing to the lists covered in **Part Two**.

*Never, ever send subscription business to an entire mailing list. It is a sure way to annoy hundreds of people who would otherwise like to like you. Always send subscribe and unsubscribe messages to the list's administrative address.*

You will usually receive an automated response to your subscription request detailing any list rules, helpful hints, and useful list commands. Save these messages! You'll find them indispensable when you're in a rush

## How to Get on and off E-Mail Discussion Lists

**M**ailing lists on the Internet use several different programs for their administration. The commands and syntax for subscribing and managing your subscription can vary. The following commands will get you on and off the lists. List programs usually send you a confirming message with an explanation of other useful commands, including the digest command and commands for accessing the list archives. If you didn't get one (or lost it), send a help message to the list administrative address. Automated list programs ignore the subject line, so you don't need to use one. Internet mailing lists with names such as list-request@wherever.edu are often managed by a real person. A subject line may make that person's life easier.

*Remember,* send subscription business to the list's administrative address (that is, to listproc@whereever.edu), *not* to the list distribution address (that is, to health@whereever.edu).

**To subscribe:**

Listserv and Listproc: Subscribe *LIST-NAME Yourfirstname Yourlastname*

Mailserv: Subscribe *listname*

Majordomo: Subscribe *listname*

**To get a list of commands:**

All programs: help

**To get off a list:**

All programs: Unsubscribe *listname*

to go on vacation, need to switch to a digest form of the list, or want to unsubscribe because the list has wandered hopelessly off topic.

## INTERNET NEWSGROUPS

If e-mail is the heart of the Internet's circulatory system, *newsgroups*—also known as Usenet news, net news, and network news—are its soul. That may sound like hyperbole, but newsgroups are a vast, sprawling (and sometimes brawling) town square in cyberspace with a foment of ideas and interchange. Newsgroups are electronic discussion groups, often likened to bulletin boards where you read what others write and post on a topic and where you can post your own thoughts.

Newsgroups are organized into hierarchies by topic family. (The list in Table 1.2 covers hierarchies used in this book. For a complete list, see a standard Internet reference.) Hierarchies are divided into *mainstream hierarchies*, which have been extensively screened and are carried by most providers, and *alternative hierarchies*, including the alt hierarchy itself where just about anything goes. The volume of news has increased dramatically (thousands of newsgroups and growing), so not all Internet sites carry all newsgroups. Because some groups carry material that is not "family oriented," some sites eliminate those as well. Newsgroups vary in tone and content. A sizable number cover health and fitness issues, including support groups for a number of illnesses and chronic conditions and online self-help groups concerned with emotional issues.

| Table 1.2 Newsgroup Hierarchies | |
|---|---|
| news. | About Usenet news. |
| rec. | Recreational newsgroups. |
| misc. | Newsgroups that don't fit the other topics. |
| sci. | Scientific discussions. |
| alt. | Newsgroups outside the main hierarchies. Cover a range of topics. |

## NEWSREADER PROGRAMS

Your choice of newsreader programs depends a lot on what your provider offers; most public access systems have one or more Unix newsreader—*rn, trn, nn,* or *tin.* If you're running on a big system or have SLIP/PPP access, a client program will manage your news.

## SUBSCRIBING, UNSUBSCRIBING, POSTING, AND NAVIGATING

All newsreaders perform a few basic functions: signing you onto and off the newsgroup, helping you put in your two cents' worth, and moving around the newsgroups. These are important functions, because you can quickly feel overwhelmed among thousands of groups and a lot of traffic.

All these programs set up a news file for you that tracks the groups you've subscribed to, the articles you've read, and so on. In your initial sign-on for news, you'll need to indicate which of the available set of newsgroups you want to read. This can take a while! Most offer you the option of checking for more new newsgroups (and it seems like there are *always* more) at sign-in thereafter.

If you have a "point-and-click" newsreader client program, you'll read and post news in a familiar Windows-like environment (see Figure 1.8), using your mouse to select messages to read, skip, and discard. If you have a dial-up account, though, you may need to learn to use one of the Unix newsreader programs.

The Unix newsreaders are fairly intuitive for basic use. You always press the spacebar to respond to the default for whatever task is before you, whether it is moving to the next group or reading the next page. Most Unix newsreaders have several commands in common. (Table 1.3 shows a selected list of newsreader commands that work in some common Unix

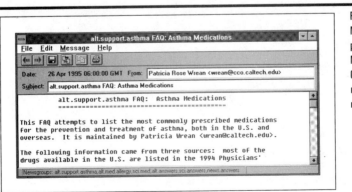

Figure 1.8:
Newsreader client programs, such as NewtNews in Internet Chameleon, make managing your news-reading simple.

newsreader programs. For a complete list, check any standard Internet reference or see your provider's Help information.) Try to limit your subscriptions to a few groups until you get the feel of your newsreader program; otherwise, you may get overwhelmed and miss the fun.

### Table 1.3 Basic Newsreader Commands

| To | Command |
|---|---|
| Unsubscribe | u |
| See next page or newsgroup | spacebar |
| Quit | q |
| Post follow-up article | f |
| Get help | h |
| Get manual | man *newsreadername* |

*Lurk first. Lurkers are those who read a mailing list or newsgroup without contributing. It's nothing to be ashamed of, and in fact it's a real virtue for new members. Listen and learn for a few weeks at least before you send in your first message.*

## FILE TRANSFER PROTOCOL (FTP)

The Internet's File Transfer Protocol (FTP) is a tool that you use to transfer files from one Internet-connected computer to another. You most often use FTP to access the huge repositories of public files on the Net. Systems around the world make their archives available to outside users.

For example, you can use FTP to download a document about nutrition in pregnancy that we found in an archie search. If you have a client program, you would enter the information in the program's FTP dialog boxes and then select the files from the server system to be downloaded to your computer (see Figure 1.9).

If you are using a dial-up Unix account, your FTP request is sent one command at a time. Basically, it goes like this:

**1.** From your system prompt, type ftp rtfm.mit.edu julian.uwo.ca.

**2.** When you are asked for Name, type anonymous.

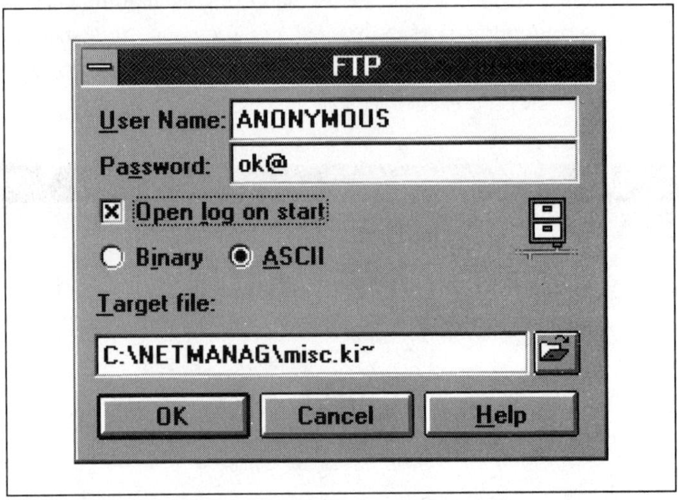

Figure 1.9:
An FTP client program
will automatically
fetch files from the
computer where
they're archived.

**3.** The next prompt will ask for a password, usually your e-mail address; so type youremailaddress.

**4.** Use the cd (change directory) command to get to the right directory by typing

cd./pub/usenet-by-groups/misc-kids/pregnancy/bradley/

**5.** Tell the host that you want the document "Nutrition," with the command

get nutrition

**6.** When you're done, at the ftp> prompt, type quit.

Here's how your FTP session would look. What you type is in **boldface**.

**% ftp julian.uwo.ca rtfm.mit.edu**
Connected to julian.uwo.ca rtfm.mit.edu
220 julian.uwo.ca rftm.mit.edu ftp server ready
Name: **anonymous**
331 Guest login ok, send ident as password.

Password: *youremailaddress*
230 Guest login ok, access restrictions apply.
ftp> **cd doc/FAQ/misc-kids/pregnancy/bradley/**
**cd /pub/usenet-by-groups/misc-kids/pregnancy/**
250 CWD command successful.
ftp> **get nutrition**
200 PORT command successful.
150 Opening data connection for nutrition (4411 bytes).
ftp> **quit**
221 Goodbye.

The nutrition in pregnancy document will then appear in your directory on your Internet system. If you're using a dial-up Internet connection, you'll still have to download the file to get it on your system at home.

## Which Tools Do What?

It's easy to get confused about the basic Internet tools and what they do. Here's the nutshell version.

- **archie** searches for files in public computer archives. After he finds them, you'll need FTP to bring them home.

- **File Transfer Protocol** (FTP) lets you move files from one system to another. For example, you use FTP to transfer files from public computer archives to your own system.

- **Gopher** is a navigating system that organizes participating Internet resources into easy-to-use menu systems and links them together. Gopher has some basic facilities for getting information, in the form of documents usually, back to your home system.

- **Telnet** is the tool that lets you log into the public spaces on other computers to get information or use their resources.

- **Veronica** is a search tool for Gopher resources.

# USING TELNET

Telnet is the Internet tool that lets you log in to other computers on the Net, no matter where you are. You can use Telnet to access your private account on a remote system (if you're working away from home, for example) or to access publicly available resources on systems around the country. You can reach many Telnet resources on health and fitness through Gopher systems, but if you don't have Gopher access, you can get to many of them through Telnet alone.

> *Telnet itself is simple to use. Although it has a number of commands, you'll probably use only one or two of them for almost everything.*

Telnet itself is simple to use. Although it has a number of commands, you'll probably use only one or two of them for almost everything. To access a remote system, type the command telnet followed by the resource address *hostname.domain*. If the system is public, you'll be greeted with instructions for using it and given any information necessary for logging in. At this point, note the commands you'll need to log off the remote system.

The only complicated thing about using Telnet is that once you activate the telnet command, you leave your home system and use another computer, which may interpret keystrokes and commands differently from those on your home system. Most are standardized, however, so Telnet use becomes almost transparent.

When you're ready to end your Telnet session, follow the log-off routine for the remote system. If you get stuck, try typing ctrl-]; this key combination should get you back to your host system. If you see the prompt telnet>, type quit, and you'll be back home again.

# Internet Navigators and Search Tools

As the Internet has gotten bigger and as the number of publicly available resources has grown, the Internet community has responded with more and better tools to navigate the Internet and seek out its resources. Tools such as Gopher and WWW have helped link resources; so you can travel almost effortlessly from one computer and resource to another. Search tools such as archie for FTP archives, Veronica for Gopherspace, and WAIS, Lycos, and WebCrawler for the WWW help you track down information.

## SEARCHING WITH ARCHIE

You can use archie to search the public anonymous FTP archives for files by name but, unfortunately, not for file contents. You may have an archie client program on your own system, if you have direct or SLIP/PPP access, or your access provider may have an archie client loaded on its system. Even if you don't have access to an archie client, you can Telnet to a public archie server. Table 1.4 shows only a few of the public archie servers. For a complete list,

| Table 1.4 Archie Server Locations | |
| --- | --- |
| **Location** | **Address** |
| Maryland | archie.sura.net |
| New Jersey | archie.internic.net |
| Montreal, Canada | archie.cs.mcgill.ca |
| Nebraska | archie.unl.edu |
| Japan | archie.wide.ad.jp |

check a standard Internet reference or Telnet to one of these sites and at the command line, type servers.

Even though archie has a range of commands to help you refine searches, a simply constructed search command will probably be enough to get you going. If you have a client program, simply enter the search term and select any applicable options (see Figure 1.10); the client program does the rest for you.

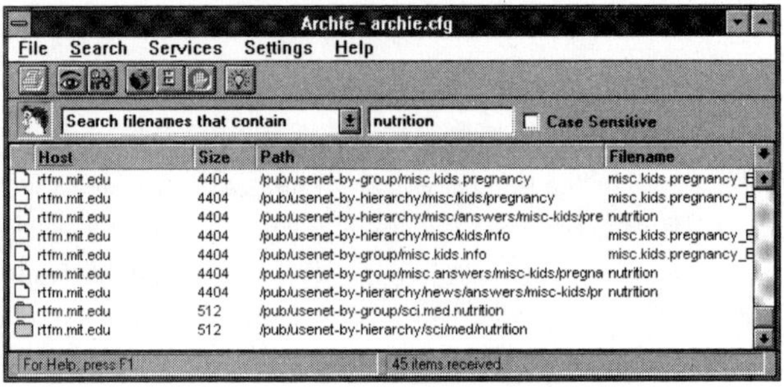

Figure 1.10:
An archie client program makes it easy to search FTP archives for files of interest.

If you are using a dial-up account and don't have access to an archie client program, you'll need to access a public archie server. Here's what you do:

**1.** Telnet to the nearest archie server by typing telnet archie.*hostname.domain.*

**2.** Log in as instructed.

**3.** Tell archie what you want to search for by typing find *yoursearchterm*

**4.** Wait for archie to respond with matches it finds. You can then use anonymous FTP to retrieve the files that most closely match your search term.

Here's how your search would look. What you type is in **boldface**.

% **telnet archie.sura.net cs.mcgill.ca**

Welcome to archie!

archie-> **find nutrition**

\# Search type: exact

working. .

Host rtfm.mit.edu

last updated 08:00:00 12 Mar 1995

Location: /pub/usenet-by-hierarchy/sci/med

DIRECTORY drwxrwxr-x 512 bytes 20:10 8 Mar 1995 /pub/usenet-by-hierarchy/sci/med/
   nutrition

Host rtfm.mit.edu

last updated 08:00:00 12 Mar 1995

Location: /pub/usenet-by-group/misc.answers/misc-kids/pregnancy/bradley/nutrition

Directory -rw-rw-r— 4404 bytes  /pub/usenet-by-group/misc.answers/
   misc-kids/pregnancy/bradley/nutrition

Host julian.uwo.ca.

Last updated 10:07 8 Mar 1995

Location: /doc/FAQ/misc-kids/pregnancy/bradley/

FILE -rwxr-xr-x 4411 bytes 18:35: 13 Feb 1995 nutrition

archie-> **quit**

If you expect to do a lot of archie searching, you can learn more about archie's other commands from any standard Internet reference book.

# SEARCHING WITH GOPHER

Gopher is a terrific Internet navigator that organizes resources into simple, straightforward menus. It eliminates the need to track dozens of Telnet and FTP resource addresses, and it lets you tunnel through the Internet to connect with thousands of Gopher sites around the world (see Figure 1.11).

Most access systems offer Gopher, and if you have direct access, you'll likely have a nifty Gopher client program. The only disadvantage is that the main menus of Gopher servers have become so large, with so many systems on board, that they are difficult to browse. And, of course, Gopher's famed tunneling effect sometimes leaves you wondering where you are or where you've been.

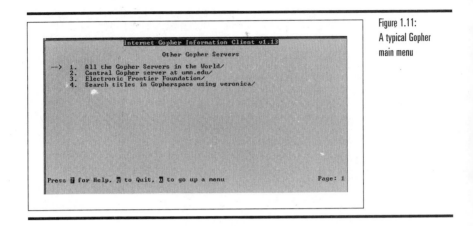

Figure 1.11:
A typical Gopher
main menu

At its simplest, Gopher is a cinch to use, but don't let its simplicity belie its power. You select entries from menus by entering the menu number or by navigating the menus with your mouse or cursor keys (see Figure 1.12). Menus are "nested," sometimes several layers deep, and when you select an item that is on another computer, Gopher will send you off to another host without your really ever knowing.

Gopher has commands, among others (see Table 1.5), to download documents or files directly or to e-mail them back to your own computer. (Table 1.5 shows a partial list of Gopher commands. For more, see a standard Internet reference.) A bookmark feature lets you mark your favorite resources for quick return trips.

```
        ┌──────────────────────────────────────────────────┐
        │        Internet Gopher Information Client v1.13   │
        │              All the Gopher Servers in the World  │
        │                                                   │
        │   2125. University of Missouri - Columbia <Mizzou1>/
        │   2126. University of Missouri - St. Louis/
        │   2127. University of Missouri - System Offices/
        │   2128. University of Missouri-Columbia -- Psychology Department/
        │   2129. University of Missouri-Kansas City/
        │   2130. University of Missouri-Rolla/
        │   2131. University of Montana/
        │ -> 2132. University of Montana Student Health Services HEALTHLINE/
        │   2133. University of Natal <Durban>/
        │   2134. University of Natal, Durban <ZA> - Elec.Eng./
        │   2135. University of Nebraska - Lincoln Computer Science & Engineering/
        │   2136. University of Nebraska at Omaha Library Gopher/
        │   2137. University of Nebraska, Omaha/
        │   2138. University of Nebraska-Lincoln  Libraries/
        │   2139. University of Nebraska-Lincoln  NU Frontier <CWIS>/
        │   2140. University of Nebraska-Lincoln Institute of Ag. & Natural Resourc
        │   2141. University of Nebraska-Lincoln Weather gopher server/
        │   2142. University of Nevada/
        │ Press @ for Help, @ to Quit, @ to go up a menu        Page: 119/1
        └──────────────────────────────────────────────────┘
```

Figure 1.12:
If you go one level
deeper to "All the
Gopher Servers in
the World," one page
(of 113 pages) looks
like this.

## Table 1.5 Basic Gopher Commands

| To | Command |
| --- | --- |
| Get a list of Gopher commands | ? |
| Go up one menu level | u |
| Go to the next page | spacebar or + |
| Go to the previous page | - |
| Get information about a menu item | = |
| Save an item to a file | s |
| Mail an item | m |
| Download an item | d |
| Add a bookmark | A |
| View your bookmark list | V |

# SEARCHING WITH VERONICA

Veronica is Gopher's search tool; Veronica is to Gopherspace what archie is to the FTP archives. Veronica will search all the Gopher menus for items or titles that contain the search term you specify.

Virtually every Gopher has a menu item for Search titles in Gopherspace using veronica/ (see Figure 1.13). When you select the menu, you'll see another menu with choices of where and how you can run your Veronica search, a document on how to compose good Veronica queries, and the Veronica FAQ.

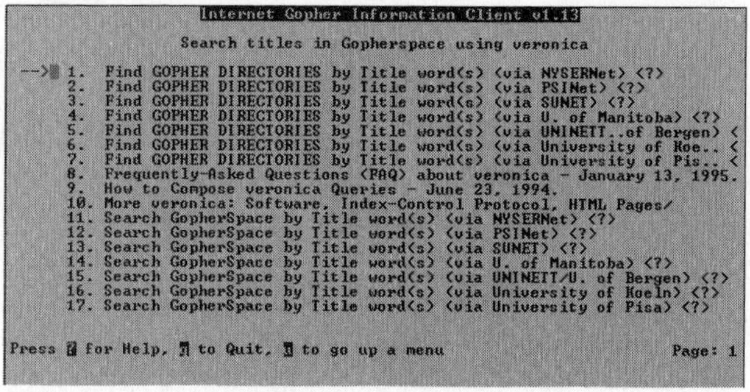

Figure 1.13:
A Veronica menu in Gopher

```
                    Internet Gopher Information Client v1.13
                   Search titles in Gopherspace using veronica
   -->  1.  Find GOPHER DIRECTORIES by Title word(s) (via NYSERNet) <?>
         2.  Find GOPHER DIRECTORIES by Title word(s) (via PSINet) <?>
         3.  Find GOPHER DIRECTORIES by Title word(s) (via SUNET) <?>
         4.  Find GOPHER DIRECTORIES by Title word(s) (via U. of Manitoba) <?>
         5.  Find GOPHER DIRECTORIES by Title word(s) (via UNINETT..of Bergen) <
         6.  Find GOPHER DIRECTORIES by Title word(s) (via University of Koe.. <
         7.  Find GOPHER DIRECTORIES by Title word(s) (via University of Pis.. <
         8.  Frequently-Asked Questions (FAQ) about veronica - January 13, 1995.
         9.  How to Compose veronica Queries - June 23, 1994.
        10.  More veronica: Software, Index-Control Protocol, HTML Pages/
        11.  Search GopherSpace by Title word(s) (via NYSERNet) <?>
        12.  Search GopherSpace by Title word(s) (via PSINet) <?>
        13.  Search GopherSpace by Title word(s) (via SUNET) <?>
        14.  Search GopherSpace by Title word(s) (via U. of Manitoba) <?>
        15.  Search GopherSpace by Title word(s) (via UNINETT/U. of Bergen) <?>
        16.  Search GopherSpace by Title word(s) (via University of Koeln) <?>
        17.  Search GopherSpace by Title word(s) (via University of Pisa) <?>

   Press ? for Help, q to Quit, u to go up a menu                    Page: 1
```

When you select a site for your search, you'll get a simple screen in which you type your search term (see Figure 1.14). Press Enter and wait for results as Veronica chugs through Gopherspace looking for your term. Veronica's results come in the form of a Gopher menu. You can add the ones you like to your bookmark list for future reference.

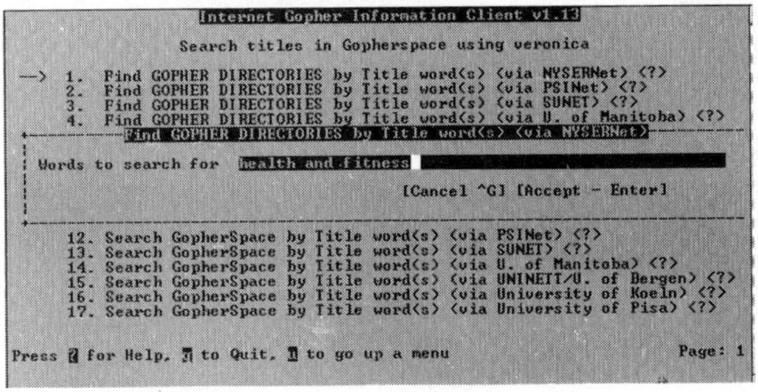

```
              Internet Gopher Information Client v1.13
             Search titles in Gopherspace using veronica
   --> 1.  Find GOPHER DIRECTORIES by Title word(s) (via NYSERNet) (?)
       2.  Find GOPHER DIRECTORIES by Title word(s) (via PSINet) (?)
       3.  Find GOPHER DIRECTORIES by Title word(s) (via SUNET) (?)
       4.  Find GOPHER DIRECTORIES by Title word(s) (via U. of Manitoba) (?)
       .........Find GOPHER DIRECTORIES by Title word(s) (via NYSERNet).........
   ! Words to search for  health and fitness                                   !
   !                                                                           !
   !                              [Cancel ^G] [Accept - Enter]                 !
   .............................................................................
      12.  Search GopherSpace by Title word(s) (via PSINet) (?)
      13.  Search GopherSpace by Title word(s) (via SUNET) (?)
      14.  Search GopherSpace by Title word(s) (via U. of Manitoba) (?)
      15.  Search GopherSpace by Title word(s) (via UNINETT/U. of Bergen) (?)
      16.  Search GopherSpace by Title word(s) (via University of Koeln) (?)
      17.  Search GopherSpace by Title word(s) (via University of Pisa) (?)

   Press ? for Help, q to Quit, u to go up a menu              Page: 1
```

Figure 1.14: Veronica is ready to search for Gopher menus that contain the words *health* and *fitness*.

# WORLD WIDE WEB (WWW)

The World Wide Web (WWW) is getting all the Net spotlight these days, and for good reason. The development of WWW *browser* software has meant that, after years of text-based, unintuitive interfaces, an easy-to-use, graphical interface is available to Internet users.

As does Gopher, WWW connects Internet resources in a seamless continuum. The difference is that WWW uses hypertext links and has the potential to join text, graphics, sound, and even video into a single viewable unit. WWW resources on the Net are growing by leaps and bounds, and WWW is an excellent resource for health-related information.

To use WWW, and here's the big drawback, you need either a direct Internet connection or a SLIP/PPP connection to the Net, a reasonably fast modem and computer, and some WWW browser software (see Figure 1.15).

Because most Internet users have dial-up access and aren't directly connected to the Net, they're essentially left out of most of the excitement. They do have some options though. Many dial-up providers offer a text-based WWW browser called lynx. Some new shareware and commercial programs (SLIPKnot and TIA, the Internet Adapter) are also beginning to bridge the

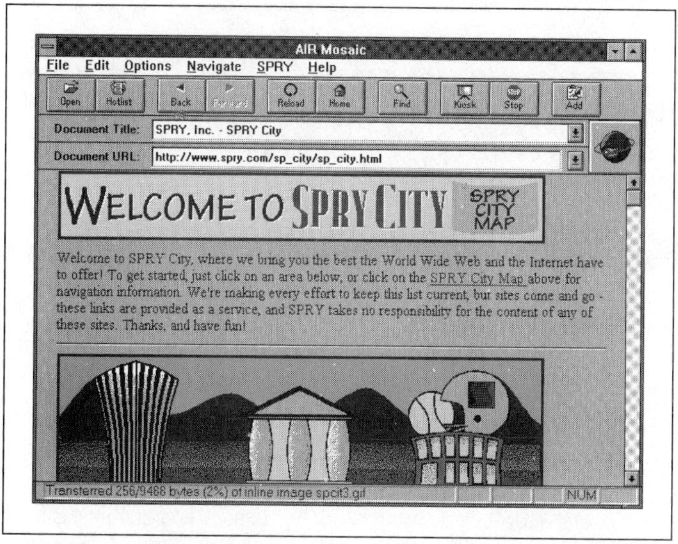

Figure 1.15:
Spry's Air Mosaic is one of the commercially available WWW browsers.

WWW gap for dial-up users. Some commercial online services are adding Internet WWW browsers, and the commercial access providers are packaging WWW browser software suites with preconfigured SLIP/PPP connections. None of these will likely be as economical as the old-fashioned shell account, but the pay-off may be worth it.

How do you use the WWW? Once you have the software, it couldn't be easier. WWW resources are identified by URLs that begin with *http://*. Your browser will have a spot for you to type the URL of the WWW site you want to start with—and off you go (see Figure 1.16).

Once you're Web-borne, you can keep clicking your mouse on interesting links and documents to see where they take you. WWW links can be files, Gophers, documents, you name it. Browsers allow you retrace your steps and to track your favorites through *hot lists* or *bookmarks*.

# WIDE AREA INFORMATION SERVER (WAIS)

The Wide Area Information Server (WAIS) is a tool that will search databases on the Internet at a greater level of depth than archie or Veronica. WAIS is a powerful tool, but it's not always simple to use. You can access a public WAIS client through Telnet (see Table 1.6) by logging in as wais. You can also

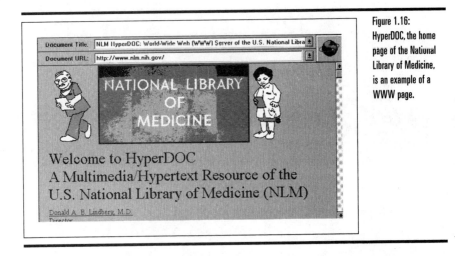

Figure 1.16:
HyperDOC, the home
page of the National
Library of Medicine,
is an example of a
WWW page.

access a public WAIS client through Gopher (which is probably easier for beginners) and through the WWW. There are also some good WAIS client programs for Windows and Unix.

To use WAIS, you first specify the *source,* which is a collection of data, you want to search. Next you enter your search terms, called *keywords* in WAIS, and press Enter to begin the search. WAIS returns you a list of all documents that contain your keywords. WAIS also gives you a *relevance score* (the highest score indicates the document that contains the most keyword matches). At this point you can look at an item or move to another search.

WAIS is a bit too complicated to illustrate in a book of this size and scope. You can try it by telnetting to one of the public WAIS clients listed below (see Table 1.6) or by using a simpler version of it in Gopher (select the menu item "WAIS Based Information") or WWW (many WWW sites offer WAIS searching).

## Table 1.6 Public WAIS Clients

| Address | Location |
| --- | --- |
| quake.think.com | Thinking Machines, Massachusetts |
| nnsc.nsf.net | NSF, Massachusetts |
| info.funet.fi | FUNET, Finland |

# REACHING RESOURCES VIA E-MAIL

What if you have only e-mail access to the Internet? Are you left out of all these great tools and resources? Fortunately not. E-mail is still a good tool for accessing some other kinds of Internet resources. In fact, almost every other Internet tool has a way for e-mail-only users to access those resources. Even if you have a boatful of Internet tools and navigators, e-mail access is often a convenient way to search for information and get the relevant documents without spending a lot of time wandering around online. FTP, archie, Gopher, WAIS, and WWW all have mail servers.

If you're interested in using these Internet tools by e-mail, send an e-mail message to one of the addresses in Table 1.7, and include a help command in the body of the message. The mail servers will send you an information document with instructions and commands.

| Table 1.7 Internet Tools and Resources via E-Mail | | | |
|---|---|---|---|
| **Internet Tool/Resource** | **Mailserver Address** | **Help Address** | **Help Message** |
| archie | archie@archie.cs.mcgill.ca | same | help |
| Ftpmail | bitftp@pucc.princeton.edu | same | help |
| Gophermail | Gophermail@calvin.edu | Gopher@calvin.edu | help |
| WAISmail | waismail@quake.think.com | same | help |
| WWW e-mail Browser | listserv@mail.w3.org | same | www |

Now that you know how to get *to* the Internet and how to get around when you're there, it's time to begin the journey. Move ahead to **Part Two** to see what's out there on the Internet for health and fitness resources.

# Part Two: Health and Fitness Travel Guide

# Being Well, Staying Well

What does it take to stay healthy these days? It seems as though the news is filled every week with stories of research studies telling us we need to do *more* of this or eat *less* of that. Whatever the current fad or flurry, the basics of taking care of ourselves will stay with us: maintain a healthy lifestyle, exercise and enjoy life, eat well and moderately, take care of the ailments and illnesses that come our way, and keep a positive mental attitude. Easier said than done, isn't it?

Fortunately, a lot of help and support is out there. What follows is some of the wealth of resources on health and fitness we've found on the Internet. Whether they're one-page documents, links of networked resources, or e-mail or newsgroup discussion lists, they have something interesting to offer.

## THE ONLINE HEALTH REFERENCE SHELF

Every home bookshelf is anchored by a few good reference books. On the Internet, the equivalent resources cover a number of topics or help you search out more specific information.

### The Medical List: Internet Clinical Medicine Resources

gopher://una.hh.lib.umich.edu:70/00/inetdirsstacks/medclin:malet

The Medical List is maintained by Gary Malet, MD, and Lee Hancock, two specialists in finding and tracking medical information on the Internet. The Medical List is a comprehensive catalog of clinical information that cuts across the whole medical spectrum. If you're looking for resources on a topic not included in this book, the Medical List is a good place to begin. It is updated periodically to include new resources.

A Web version of the Medical List, called Medical Matrix-Guide to Internet Medical Resources (see Figure 2.1), is available at

http://kuhttp.cc.ukans.edu/cwis/units/medcntr/Lee/HOMEPAGE.HTML

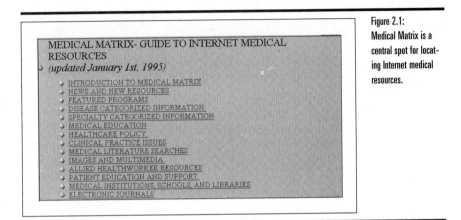

Figure 2.1:
Medical Matrix is a central spot for locating Internet medical resources.

## Yahoo Internet Resources

http://www.yahoo.com/Health

Yahoo is a searchable index of Internet resources. It has a good set of links to big collections of health resources, some of which are included elsewhere in this book. You can use Yahoo to keyword search by topic or to quickly link to health resources. The menu runs from Alternative Medicine to Women's Health and includes items such as Computer-Related Health Hazards, Dentistry, Insurance, Pharmacology, and lots more. This index is a great place to start any search for Internet health-related information. In fact, there's so much at Yahoo, you may never get around to visiting any other resource!

## Health and Medicine in the News

gopher://lenti.med.umn.edu:71/11/news

Have you ever read a newspaper report on some medical breakthrough and wanted to get more detailed information? Or wondered about the science behind the news? The Health and Medicine in the News section of the Bio-Medical Library at the University of Minnesota's Gopher has taken a nifty approach to answering those questions. The library scans a major daily newspaper in the Minneapolis/Saint Paul area for health-related articles that announce new research findings and refer to an upcoming article in a scholarly journal. The references to the news article briefly describe the content, cite the published literature referenced in the article, and list the results of a brief search of the recent journal literature for related references. Article entries go back to May 1994.

For example, one entry announced a new study published in the *Journal of the American Medical Association (JAMA)* that proved a heart benefit from even short bits of exercise, such as walking, gardening, or stair-climbing, scattered throughout the day. (An important boost for those of us who can't get to those 20-minute-plus aerobic workouts!) In addition to the article synopsis, the entry referenced the original article in *JAMA*—so you could look it up yourself.

# Healthwise

http://www.columbia.edu/cu/healthwise/

The Healthwise Web site and Go Ask Alice! are provided by the Columbia University Health Services and are packed with good, easy-to-understand information on a variety of health topics. The site includes the Healthwise newsletter on health issues of interest to a college community and Go Ask Alice! where you can ask health-related questions (see Figure 2.2). Alice posts the answers publicly, but the questioner remains anonymous. All answers are in a searchable archive, in date order and by topic. Alice's archives are a gold mine of solid information on topics such as nutrition and healthy diet, general health and emotional well-being, and concerns about drugs, alcohol, sex, and relationships (see Figure 2.3).

We found good information on eczema, a great bit on bread dough conditioners (ever wonder what they are?), and even a piece on the fat in refried beans. Alice, who is really a group of professional and peer health educators, appears to have impeccable credentials. Her answers are well researched, thorough, and easy to understand.

Figure 2.2:
Go Ask Alice! will
answer your health
questions ...

# Healthwise

**Healthwise** is the Health Education and Wellness program of Columbia University Health Service. We are a team of professional and peer educators committed to helping you make choices that will contribute to your personal health and happiness, the well-being of others, and to the planet we share.

Healthwise highlights--Spring 1995

Healthwise highlights--Fall 1994

Go Ask Alice!- An Interactive Question & Answer Health Line

| Go Ask Alice | /usr/local/lib/www/data/cu |
|---|---|
| /cu/healthwise | |
| on | nutrition |
| 20 | 30 |

Words to search for:

Search

Figure 2.3:
... or she'll search her
archives for health top-
ics of interest to you.

General Health

*About Alice.*

The following facility allows you to ask Alice anonymously only if your WorldWide Web browser supports HTML forms. If it does not, please ask Alice anonymously via ColumbiaNet.

Ask Alice about relationships, nutrition and diet, drugs, sex, alcohol, stress, etc.

Questions are anonymous; answers will be posted.

| false | alice@columbia.edu |
|---|---|
| Alice query | |

Go Ask Alice.

Alice,

**Please tell me whether refried beans are a healthy diet choice or not?**

Submit Question    Clear Question

*It's only fair, since Alice's services are for Columbia students, to check the archives for answers to your concerns before you blast off your own query. And remember, this service is for a college student audience, so don't be offended if some topics are a bit racier than you think they ought to be. Part of Alice's mission is to answer the questions people might be too embarrassed to ask in person.*

# Health Information, Rice University

gopher://riceinfo.rice.edu:70/11/Safety/HealthInfo

A campus health service at Rice University in Houston, Texas, this Gopher has lots of health information to interest students and nonstudents. Although a few menu items are specific to Rice, most will appeal to a much wider audience. Topics include women's health, preventive medicine, food and health, HIV/AIDS, injuries and accidents, sexually transmitted diseases, sports medicine, illness, and travel. There's even a menu item for "Texas critters that bite," just in case you have an interest in fire ants or squirrel bites.

Useful documents include those on the common cold and migraine headaches, among many others. You can get a "Stop Smoking" handout, take a cholesterol quiz, or read "The Darker Side of Tanning," about preventing skin cancer. There's a good section on sports medicine and a connection to the USDA food-labeling information regulations, which also includes information on calcium and osteoporosis, sodium and hypertension, and health claims for various nutrients.

# Health Information, University of Illinois at Urbana-Champaign

gopher:/gopher.uiuc.edu/Campus Info/Campus Services/Health Services/ Health Information

The college health services Gopher at UIUC has an extensive menu selection, including Diseases and Conditions, Nutrition, Sexuality, Stress, Tests, Women's Health, and Medications. Nested in these menus are some good patient education fact sheets on a range of topics. Some we checked out included "Sun Damage," "Allergic Rhinitis" (aka hay fever), "Overweight or Overfat?" and "Chicken Pox." They're all thorough and clearly written, and some cited background information in medical journals.

## HEALTH AND WELLNESS

The Internet has some good resources on staying healthy and getting to and maintaining a healthy lifestyle. Here are some places to look for information on fitness and wellness.

## Fitness and Exercise Discussion

FIT-L

listserv@etsuadmn.etsu.edu

For fitness and exercise discussions, the FIT-L discussion list really can't be beat. If you want to find out how to get the slipperiness back into your exercise slide, if you want tips on tightening those abs, or if you just want some motivational support for exercising after a tiring day of work and kids, sign up for this list. The quality of the conversation and the information is high. At least some of the regulars appear to be trainers, physicians, or other sports medicine professionals; many of the rest must be very committed amateurs. Exercise isn't the only topic; nutrition and motivation get equal time. Some recent discussion threads ranged from prevention and treatment of shin splints to recommendations for running shoes to conquering chocolate cravings.

FIT-L is an active list with more than 500 subscribers, usually generating several messages each day and sustaining several threads of conversation. To subscribe, send e-mail to the address above with the message Subscribe-FIT-L *Yourfirstname Yourlastname.*

*Never use an auto-responder program to handle your mail while you're on vacation, unless you can be sure to exclude mailing list messages from the automatic responses. The polite thing to do is to unsubscribe until you return or use the nomail command if it's available.*

## Fitness Discussion

misc.fitness

The misc.fitness newsgroup discusses all aspects of fitness, weight training, aerobics, body building, and nutrition. You can learn from others about body-weight to body-fat ratios, about how to gain weight if you have a low body weight, about the ins and outs of aerobic exercise, about which equipment is worth buying, and so on.

Lots of readers and posters to this group! You can get the FAQ for the misc.fitness from ftp://ftp.cray.com/pub/misc.fitness.

# Wellness Letter

gopher://enews.com/Health and Medical Center/Health & Medical Periodicals

The Internet's Electronic Newsstand is an online version of the traditional newsstand where you can browse current issues of a whole raft of magazines and journals. The Electronic Newsstand goes one better with searchable archives of tables of contents of back issues and featured articles, and, of course, you can use the Electronic Newsstand to easily order a subscription of the hard-copy version. Newsstand publishers put up the table of contents and one or more featured articles from each current issue.

The Wellness Letter, just one of the health-related periodicals on the Electronic Newsstand, is a well-respected monthly newsletter published by the School of Public Health at the University of California at Berkeley. The Wellness Letter features news and practical advice on preventive medicine and healthy living. Recent articles posted on the Electronic Newsstand included "Wellness Tips," an interesting piece on the placebo effect called "The Power of Hope," and a "Food for Thought Quiz." (Did you know that pink grapefruit has 40 times the beta carotene of white grapefruit?) The Electronic Newsstand version of the Wellness Letter makes for some good online browsing.

# Health in Perspective Newsletter

sample@perspective.com

The Health in Perspective Newsletter is one of the new commercial ventures on the Net, as is the Electronic Newsstand mentioned earlier. Both offer a service and also keep to the Internet's mission of sharing information. Health in Perspective is a monthly that publishes consumer-level news and research on health, nutrition, and lifestyle. Articles are heavily weighted toward healthy diet (as defined by recent research) and toward heart disease and cancer-risk reduction. Many articles discuss recent research in plain language, but don't, unfortunately, always cite the professional literature.

You can get a free sample issue by sending e-mail to the address above with the message sample-request. Subscriptions are modestly priced.

# PREVENTIVE CARE

It may sound a bit trite, but an ounce of prevention *is* worth a pound of cure. Staying healthy is a lot easier than recovering from illness or injury. Here are some Internet resources on preventive care.

## Clinical Preventive Services

gopher://gopher.nlm.nih.gov/11/hstat/guide_cps

http://text.nlm.nih.gov/cps/www/cps.html

The U.S. Department of Health and Human Services has sponsored the Clinical Preventive Services (CPS) Task Force to review and recommend preventive care for common health problems. The CPS documents cover prevention and screening guidelines for dozens of conditions, from high blood pressure to various forms of cancer to depression. Although written for a medical audience, the guidelines are relatively easy to read and contain a balanced presentation of the task force members' review of current practice and research. Relevant research citations are included in each screening guideline. The guidelines also include recommendations for immunizations, preventive drug therapies, health-behavior counseling, and schedules for physical examinations

## Cardiac Health Discussion

CARDIAC-PREV

mailserv@ac.dal.ca

The CARDIAC-PREV discussion list is devoted to the prevention of heart disease through, as the statement of purpose says, "non-pharmacological means." The list covers the obvious—diet, exercise, and smoking—but is also open to discussing the economic, social, educational, and cultural factors that contribute to heart disease. CARDIAC-PREV is a fairly low-volume list with good content. Definitely worth a look.

To subscribe, send e-mail to the address above with the message Subscribe CARDIAC-PREV. Do not include your name. A subject line is not necessary.

## Family Health

http://www.tcom.ohiou.edu:80/family-health.html

Family Health (see Figure 2.4) is a series of brief radio programs from Ohio University College of Osteopathic Medicine made available as audio files on the Family Health home page. Topics cover common health problems and concerns, for example, restless legs syndrome, vacuum cleaners and allergies, sprained ankles, stress and high blood pressure. The programs are about 2.5 minutes long; your computer must be capable of playing back files in .au format, or you'll need a program (some are in the public domain) that will convert the .au files to something your speaker can handle. Definitely worth a listen!

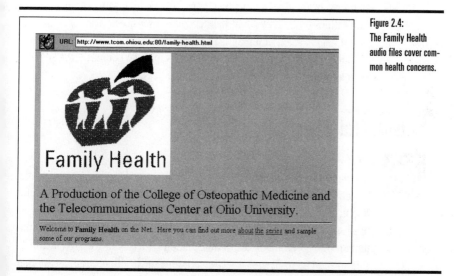

Figure 2.4:
The Family Health audio files cover common health concerns.

## Safety and Health

gopher://dewey.tis.inel.gov:2013/1

The U.S. Department of Energy (DOE) has put up a great Gopher with excellent safety-related documents on a range of topics. Although many are specific to DOE activities (you may not be too interested in crane transport safety), some—such as the ones on preventing indoor slips and falls, ladder safety, or the risk of miscarriage from electromagnetic fields—cover topics of wider interest. The menu includes Safety and Health Bulletins, Safety and Health Actions, Health Hazard Alerts, Health Watch, Safety Notes, Occupational Safety Observer, The Safety Connection, OSH Technical Reference Manual, and a search facility.

## Bike Helmet Safety

http://www.bhsi.org:80/

Bike helmets prevent untold numbers of serious head injuries every year and would prevent even more if people would wear them—and insist that their kids do so as well. Here's an Internet home for bike helmet information, sponsored by the Bike Helmet Safety Institute (BHSI), with online and print publications on helmet safety, helmet comparisons, and help for setting up a local helmet safety campaign. The BHSI also monitors mandatory helmet legislation and applicable design standards for bike helmets. This site also includes links to other Internet cycling resources.

## National Health Information Center

http://nhic-nt.health.org:80/

A service of the U.S. Office of Disease Prevention and Health Promotion, the National Health Information Center has gone online with some very helpful resources. The Online Health Information Resource Database (see Figure 2.5) has lists of toll-free numbers for health information and links to information on U.S. government health information centers, plus a search facility to sort through them. There's a section on work-site health promotion, another on national health observances, and a locator for other U.S. government health resources.

## TRAVEL HEALTH

Traveling is exciting, educational, relaxing—and no fun at all if you're sick or worried about getting sick. Here are some Net resources for staying well while you're on the move. Remember, though, no immunizations are required for travel on the Internet!

Figure 2.5:
The National Health
Information Center has
gone online to bring
you access to health
information resources.

## International Travelers Clinic

http://www.intmed.mcw.edu/travel.html

This Web page from the International Travelers Clinic at the Medical College of Wisconsin has a wealth of information on international travel, for example, required immunizations and disease hot spots around the world. Did you know that rabies is a big problem for visitors to many developing countries? Worried about the plague outbreak in India? You can get authoritative information here. Plus tips on traveling while pregnant, assembling a travel medicine kit, avoiding altitude sickness, and dealing with motion sickness. The site has links to country maps and information, to the CIA World Factbook and the U.S. State Department Travel Warnings, and to the University of Manitoba Travel Library, among others.

## Staying Healthy in Asia, Africa, and Latin America

http://www.moon.com:7000/lh/travel.health.html

This Internet resource is an abridged, online version of the book by the same name. Chapter titles include "Before You Go," "Arrival and Preventing Illness," "Diagnosis and Treatment of Illness," and "After You Return Home." You can use this resource to learn, for example, what you can drink safely and how to prevent malaria. Definitely take a look if you plan a trip to any of these areas.

## Stanford Travel Medicine Service

http://www-leland.stanford.edu:80/~naked/stms.html

This is another Web page on travel health, and a good one. It covers wilderness travel medicine and has selections on immunizations, medical kits, gastrointestinal illnesses, insect repellents, mountain sickness, malaria, and HIV. Check out the excellent fact sheet on traveling with children and keeping them healthy.

## World Health Organization International Travel and Health Information

http://www.who.ch:80/TravelAndHealth/TravelAndHealth_Home.html

Go right to the source for a country-by-country list of vaccination certification requirements and for information on immunization requirements and the geographic distribution of potential health risks for travelers (see Figure 2.6).

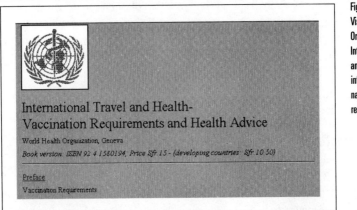

International Travel and Health-
Vaccination Requirements and Health Advice

World Health Organization, Geneva

Book version: ISBN 92 4 1580194, Price Sfr. 15.- (developing countries: Sfr. 10.50)

Preface
Vaccination Requirements

**Figure 2.6:**
Visit the World Health Organization's International Travel and Health page for information on international vaccination requirements.

# WOMEN'S HEALTH

Women have unique health and wellness concerns that often get short shrift in some venues. Not so on the Net, where there are good standard medical resources, interesting alternative therapies, and a supportive environment for online discussions.

## Women's Health Topics

http://www.mit.edu:8001/people/sorokin/women/index.html

The Women's Health section of the Women's home page covers a range of topics of interest to women. Included are a bibliography on women in science, health, and technology and links to the Breast Cancer Information Clearinghouse, the Midwifery Today Web server, and the Index of Birth-Related Information. This Web site is a good jumping-off place for all kinds of information on women's health and related issues.

## Atlanta Reproductive Health Centre

http://www.mindspring.com:80~mperloe/homepage.html

This Web page, put up by an Atlanta fertility specialist, is a good place to start a search for information on a number of women's health issues, including infertility and endometriosis. It includes links to the FAQ for Resolve, a highly regarded infertility resource and advocacy group, to the Endometriosis Association, and to WITSENDO, the e-mail discussion group for endometriosis. A complete online version of a book on infertility by the author of the page rounds out the offerings.

## Kristi's PMS Information

http://www.ccnet.com/~diatribe/pms.html

Women troubled by PMS (premenstrual syndrome) will find some interesting alternative treatments for that bedeviling condition, including herbs, vitamins, and aromatherapy. You can also link to other women's health and alternative medicine resources from this Web site.

# Menopause Discussion

MENOPAUS

listserv@psuhmc.hmc.psu.edu

The MENOPAUS list is like having a cup of afternoon tea with some good—and very well-informed—friends. Discussions concern all the issues facing women as they reach "middle age," including coping with the physical symptoms of menopause. Members talk about the advantages and disadvantages of the various hormonal/nonhormonal therapies for menopause symptoms. The group seems about evenly split between hormone replacement therapy users and those who prefer more natural interventions, such as nutritional supplements and exercise or no intervention at all. And all without a lot of controversy about which is the right path. Lively discussions concern many other topics, including the state of the health-care system, emotional support, and aging, exercise, and diet. Some members are health professionals, and the information content of the list seems as good as its members are friendly and supportive.

MENOPAUS is an active list, with 400-plus members and with as many as 30 messages a day. It's a good list to get in digest form if you have trouble keeping up with your mail. To subscribe, send e-mail to the address above with Subscribe MENOPAUS *Yourfirstname Yourlastname* in the body of the message. No subject line is necessary. MENOPAUS contributions are archived automatically, and you can get an index of the archives by sending the index command to the list administrative address above.

# Women's Health Electronic News Line

WMN-HLTH

listproc@u.washington.edu

The Women's Health Electronic News Line (WMN-HLTH) is an electronic newsletter and discussion list from the Center for Women's Health Research at the University of Washington in Seattle. The list content is eclectic, just about anything on the general topic of women's health goes, from discussions of calcium supplementation to contraception to the legal damage awards for faulty silicone breast implants.

To subscribe, send e-mail to the address above with the message Subscribe WMN-HLTH *Yourfirstname Yourlastname*.

*Remember that hundreds of people may read what you write, and many lists and newsgroups archive their messages!*

## SMOKING

It isn't easy to quit smoking, but just about everyone agrees that smoking isn't very compatible with a healthy lifestyle. Here are some Internet resources that might help you or a loved one finally win that battle.

## Smoke-Free Discussion

SMOKE-FREE

listproc@msstate.edu

SMOKE-FREE is an online version of a traditional smokers' support group, "a support list for people recovering from addiction to cigarettes," according to the list owner. "Anybody with an interest in quitting smoking or in helping others quit is encouraged to participate in the discussion." The long-timers share their struggles and triumphs to encourage newcomers with the shakes who are just trying to get through Day 2. Lapsed smokers are gently urged to try to quit one more time. And everyone shares tips and tricks for engaging in the battle with nicotine. Some quit with patches, some quit with nicotine substitutes such as gum, some quit cold turkey. This list also posts relevant news clips on the health and political issues of smoking and tobacco.

> ### More...
>
> Looking for other electronic discussion and support groups on smoking?
> Check out the newsgroups: alt.support.stop-smoking, alt.support.non-smokers, and alt.support.non-smokers.moderated.

To subscribe, send e-mail to the above address with Subscribe SMOKE-FREE *Yourfirstname Yourlastname* in the body of the message. No subject line is necessary.

## Smoking and Smoking Cessation

http://128.19.106.42/smoking.html

The Arizona Health Sciences Library has a nifty Web page that offers links to a range of documents, other Web pages, research indexes, and online groups that discuss smoking and quitting. Also featured are a political cartoon on the tobacco industry and a list called "The Simpsons *vs.* Smoking" that contains every incident of smoking or cigarettes on the animated TV show. Try the link to the University of Pennsylvania's <u>Smoking, Tobacco, and Cancer</u> page (or go directly to http://cancer.med.upenn.edu:80/1s/topics) for documents such as "Second Hand Smoke" and "Role of Media in Tobacco Control."

## EXERCISE GUIDELINES

We all know we should exercise, but even when we're motivated, some risks are associated with simply going ahead and not knowing what you're doing. The Internet has some good sources of exercise guidelines. Here are a few.

## Healthline, University of Montana

gopher://healthline.umt.edu:70/11/UofM/hhp

Healthline has a lot of excellent, general interest health information, including good patient education fact sheets on problems ranging from ankle sprains to stomach flu. There's a real little gold mine, though, in the Sports Medicine menu (see Figure 2.7). Wondering about the effects of the air pollution you breathe when you're exercising? Check here. Healthline also has good information on exercising at high altitudes, exercising during pregnancy, improving your performance in racquet sports, strength training for Nordic skiing, and more. One menu level above, in the General Health Information menu, is a good fact sheet, "Shaping Up Safely."

You can also get to Healthline via telnet to health.umt.edu (log in as health) or through the WWW at http://healthline.umt.edu:700.

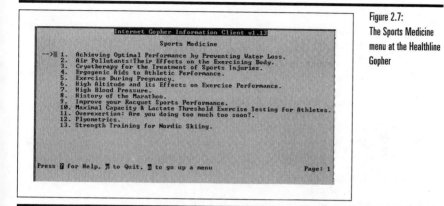

Figure 2.7:
The Sports Medicine
menu at the Healthline
Gopher

# Health Information, University of Illinois at Urbana-Champaign

gopher://gopher.uiuc.edu/Campus Info/Campus Services/Health Services/ Health Information/Fitness

The UIUC Gopher contains more good stuff. The Fitness menu has information on abdominal strengthening, improving flexibility through proper stretching, and walk/jog program progression. There's even a document titled "Are You Exercising Too Much?" that includes a scoring system to help you decide if you're overdoing it.

# Abdominal Training Questions and Answers

http:/www.dstc.edu.au:80/staff/nigel-ward/abfaq/abdominal-training.html

Here's a thorough discussion of the dos and don'ts of getting great abdominals. It's taken from the newsgroup misc.fitness. Wondering what's wrong with sit-ups? Want to get rid of that spare tire, those love handles? There's information here on structuring a routine, exercising abs during pregnancy, and more (see Figure 2.8).

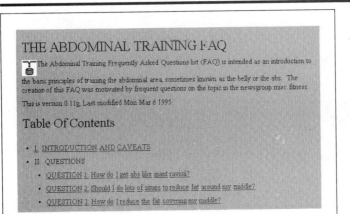

Figure 2.8:
The Abdominal FAQ
assembles years of
wisdom from the
misc.fitness newsgroup
about conditioning the
abdominal muscles.

## Health and Fitness

http://bigdipper.umd.edu/health-fitness/index.html

This Web page is big on weightlifting and also has links to FAQs on stretching and flexibility and the abdominal training FAQ mentioned above. There are links to other Internet health-related resources and to resources on female bodybuilding, weightlifting, and workout plans.

## SPORTS

Looking for sports information? The best place to start for individual sports is in the rec.sports newsgroups. Many sports aficionados have put up Gopher servers and Web pages.

### More . . .

For more Internet sports information, try some of these sports-related newsgroups:

rec.scuba
rec.skiing

rec.sport.golf
rec.sport.rowing
rec.sport.swimming
rec.sport.tennis
rec.sport.volleyball

# Global Cycling Network

gopher://cycling.org

VeloNet, the Global Cycling Network, has a Gopher with lots to interest cyclers and would-be cyclers. The menu options include bicycle organizations, ride calendars, Internet mailing lists and newsgroups devoted to cycling, pointers to other cycling resources on the Internet, and even a full WAIS search of all VeloNet documents on cycling. This is an international Gopher with resources from Australia to Europe and around the U.S. You can also get to VeloNet via the Web at http://cycling.org.

# Sports Psychology

SPORTPSY

listserv@vm.temple.edu

The SPORTPSY list is devoted to the topics of exercise and sports psychology. It's primarily a professional list, but motivated amateurs will also find much of interest here. Popular topics include motivation in sports, athletes' eating disorders, and issues that arise in counseling student athletes.

To subscribe, send e-mail to the address above with the message Subscribe SPORTPSY *Yourfirstname Yourlastname.*

# Sports Science

majordomo@stonebow.otago.ac.nz

SPORTSCI is a mailing list for serious athletes, coaches, exercise physiologists, trainers, and the like. A relatively young list, SPORTSCI covers the science of sports, including measuring physical performance, training and competing under extreme conditions—such as altitude and extreme cold and heat—diet, supplements, and other nutritional issues. This is definitely not the place for couch potatoes or weekend athletes. SPORTSCI has about 600 members. The small size and tight format make for good information and a positive collegial atmosphere.

To subscribe, send e-mail to the address above with the message SUBSCRIBE SPORTSCI.

# Women in Sports, Health, Physical Education, Recreation, and Dance

WISHPERD

listserv@sjsuvml.sjsu.edu

WISHPERD is a list for discussing anything having to do with women in any kind of athletic endeavor mentioned in its title. Discussions range from the basics to the politics of women and sports to the future of Title IX to Martina's baseball career. The traffic is moderate here, and the discussions are thoughtful.

To subscribe, send e-mail to listserv@sjsuvml.sjsu.edu with the message SUB-SCRIBE WISHPERD *Yourfirstname Yourlastname*.

# Dead Runners Society

dead-runners-society-request@uns.sas.com

Dead Runners Society (DRS) is self-described as "a discussion group for people who like to talk about running." It's an active list with more than 1000 members.

The DRS also has a Web home page (http://www.furman.edu:80/drs/drs.html) with archives of its best information on training, injuries, software to track your running, weather (How *does* humidity affect your performance?), and lists of running-related publications. The page also has links to other Internet running resources. A great resource.

To subscribe, send e-mail to the address above with Subscribe in the subject line and the message:

*Subscribe Youremailaddress.*

---

## More...

For more information on running, including race information, tips and FAQs, check out these Internet resources:

The Running Page:
http://sunsite.unc.edu:80/drears/running/running.html

rec.running newsgroup

The rec.running FAQ:
ftp://relay.cs.toronto.edu/pub/usenet/news.answers/running.faq

## Inline Skating

http://www.xs4all.nl:80/~lowlevel/skate/inline-skating.html

The Low-Level inline skating Web page has great graphics, tutorials on inline skating, a guide to inline skating terms, and links to other resources of interest. Based in Amsterdam, this page has a European slant that adds to the fun.

## Stretching and Flexibility

http://ubu.hahnemann.edu:80/Stretching/stretch.intro.html

ftp://cs.huji.ac.il/pub/doc/faq/rec/martial.arts

This is a primer on stretching and how to do it for the best effect. This document, from the rec.martial.arts FAQ, covers the physiology of stretching, flexibility, types of stretching, and how to stretch.

## Tennis Server

http://arganet.tenagra.com:80/Racquet_Workshop/Tennis.html

The Tennis Server is a terrific Web site with GIF images of tennis stars, player and equipment tips of the month, an online newsletter following the tours, shareware, and lots more. You can get the Tennis FAQ here and the Rules and Code of Tennis as well.

# Eating Well

Just about everyone agrees that eating well is important for good health. Whether you need information on nutrition basics or support for a special diet or for weight management or whether you just love to read about food and discuss food, you'll find help on the Internet.

If you're looking for something as simple as a few new recipes to expand your repertoire or as technical as information on food safety, the Internet's food and nutrition resources most likely have what you need. The land-grant colleges and universities throughout the U.S. have always had a strong interest in agriculture, food, and nutrition—and now have a strong presence on the Internet. And the U.S. government has been hard at work, as well; the Internet has offerings from the Food and Drug Administration (FDA) and the Department of Agriculture (USDA).

## THE FOOD AND NUTRITION ONLINE REFERENCE SHELF

The combination of educational, governmental, and other sites yields a treasure trove of Gophers, WWW pages, FTP, Telnet, and e-mail resources. Whatever your level of Internet access, from e-mail-only to WWW, you can access comprehensive, up-to-date, interesting, or just-plain-tasty food and nutrition resources.

## Nutrition Information

http://128.196.106.42:80/nutrition.html

The Arizona Health Sciences Library (AHSL) WWW Nutrition Guide home page is an excellent jumping-off place for finding Internet resources and information on nutrition. The Nutrition Subject Index (see Figure 2.9) has links to academic centers, including Cornell University, which has a nutrition

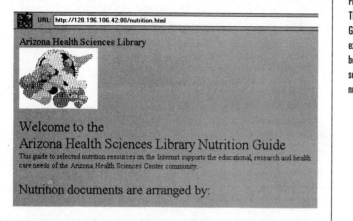

Figure 2.9:
The AHSL Nutrition Guide home page is an excellent place to begin an Internet search on food or nutrition.

database you can search. From this index you can also link to the WWW Yahoo Nutrition page and the EINet Galaxy Nutrition Index.

Check out the link to Educational Resources for brochures and teaching materials on nutrition. Other resources include grants and source information for research in agriculture and nutrition, a link to food technology sources, and another to general biomedical guides.

The Nutrient Data link has a wealth of useful information. Or you can read a document titled "The Nutrient Content of the U.S. Food Supply." Link to Veggies Unite! to search an index of more than 1500 vegetarian recipes.

# PENpages

 gopher://psupen.psu.edu

 telnet://psupen.psu.edu

PENpages, available by Gopher or Telnet from the Penn State College of Agricultural Sciences, has more than 13,000 reports, newsletters, bibliographies, and fact sheets on human nutrition, agriculture, aging, family, community development, and consumer issues.

PENpages is also home to the International Food and Nutrition (IFAN) database, a subset of PENpages that comprises documents on food and nutrition. You can search IFAN with keywords, such as specific foods (*apple*, for example), or with broader topics such as *food safety*.

 *When searching this database with two-word search terms, hyphenate them, for example, food-safety.*

So what's there? An IFAN keyword search on eating-out yielded a list of 28 articles and fact sheets, including an excellent one titled "Make Your Chinese Food Choices Heart Healthy." The regular IFAN and PENpages menus included an article that rated the accuracy of the nutrition information in various popular magazines (better to do your nutrition reading in *Cooking Light* than in *Cosmo*) and another titled "Should Children Drink Milk?" A tempting potpourri of rice recipes included a healthy one for brown rice Waldorf salad with chicken breasts (see Figure 2.10) and another for tomato-basil salad.

```
¶
·················COOL·&·CRISP·RECIPES¶
·=·=·=·=·=·=·=·=·=·=·=·=·¶
Brown·Rice·Waldorf·Salad¶
·························¶
   3/4·cup·vanilla·lowfat·yogurt¶
   1/2·cup·reduced·calorie·mayonnaise¶
   1/4·teaspoon·salt¶
   1/4·teaspoon·ground·cinnamon¶
   3·cups·cooked·brown·rice,·cooled¶
   2·medium·tart·apples,·diced¶
   1-1/4·cups·coarsely·chopped·celery¶
   1·medium·carrot,·diced¶
   3/4·cup·chopped·walnuts¶
   3/4·cup·raisins¶
   6·boneless,·skinless·chicken·breast·halves,·grilled·or·broiled¶
   Assorted·fresh·fruit·for·garnish·(optional)¶
¶
Blend·yogurt,·mayonnaise,·salt,·and·cinnamon·in·large·bowl.·Add·rice,·apples,·¶
celery,·carrot,·walnuts,·and·raisins;·mix·well.·Serve·with·grilled·chicken·¶
breasts.·Garnish·with·fresh·fruit.¶
¶
Makes·6·servings.¶
```

**Figure 2.10:** A healthy version of Waldorf salad from PENpages

The PENpages Telnet address is penpages.psu.edu. Log in with your two-letter state abbreviation (CA, for example) or log in with WORLD if you are accessing PENpages from outside the U.S. The menu structure of the Telnet version of IFAN and PENpages is a bit different from the Gopher menu, but both are straightforward and easy to use.

### International Food and Information Council

http://ificinfo.health.org:80/

The International Food and Information Council (IFIC) is a Washington, DC–based group that is funded by food and beverage industries. The council's WWW server has an interesting combination of solid nutritional information and documents supporting IFIC positions for an intended audience of consumers, teachers, and journalists. The range of documents is broad, from consumer nutrition to position papers on the Delaney Clause (the regulation that prohibits use of food additives shown to cause cancer in experimental animals) and on the use of pesticides relative to the safety of the food supply.

The consumer nutrition information is clearly written, balanced, and easy to understand. "Healthy Eating for Kids," for example, is an informative fact sheet with ten tips for kids on good nutrition. Some other family-oriented topics include teen nutrition, nutrition's role in preventing birth defects, and healthy eating during pregnancy.

# Human Nutrition (Nutrición Humana)

http://www.spin.com.mx/nutrimex/nutrimex.html

The Nutrición Humana WEB (see Figure 2.11) site in Mexico City was still under construction when we visited, but even so had plenty of operating links to useful nutrition resources. The home page is in Spanish, but most links are in English. You can find your way around easily, even if your knowledge of Spanish is slim or nonexistent. A few hints: FTP, not surprisingly, translates as FTP, and *servidores* are list servers. It's just about that easy.

And worth the trouble. The FTP section has links to FTP archives at the University of California, Irvine and to those at Oakland University. The Oakland link is home to an FTP archive of food-related software that yielded an effortless download of a software demo sampler for recipe software that, among other features, calculates the nutritional composition of your recipes. (For a look, try ftp://anonymous:oak.oakland.edu:21/SimTel/win3/food and get mcook_2.zip.)

There are plenty of links to other WWW nutrition sites and links to U.S. government resources as well. The Servidores section takes you to information on food and nutrition list servers, including DIABETIC and DIET. A section on nutrition in Mexico rounds out the offerings.

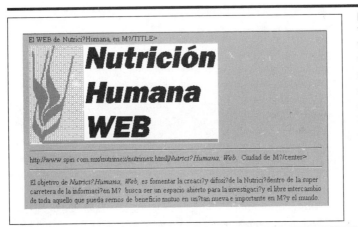

El WEB de Nutrici?Humana, en M?/TITLE>

# Nutrición Humana WEB

http://www.spin.com.mx/nutrimex/nutrimex.html]Nutrici?Humana, Web. Ciudad de M?/center>

El objetivo de *Nutrici?Humana, Web*, es fomentar la creaci?y difusi?de la Nutrici?dentro de la super carretera de la informaci?en M? busca ser un espacio abierto para la investigaci?y el libre intercambio de toda aquello que pueda sernos de beneficio mutuo en un?tan nueva e importante en M?y el mundo.

Figure 2.11:
The Nutrición Humana WEB (Human Nutrition WEB) site in Mexico City is a feast of food and nutrition links. The site's home page is in Spanish, but most links are in English.

## Security?

Security of your own system and information depends primarily on how you're connected to the Net. If you're using a dial-up system or a commercial service, your vulnerability is limited. You should run virus protection software on your own computer if you expect to download files, especially shareware, from other computers. If you're simply using e-mail, reading news, and the like, you don't have much to worry about.

Businesses on the Net are trying to improve the security of online transactions. Before you send your credit card number over the Internet, find out which protections are in place. Some e-mail encryption schemes, such as PGP (Pretty Good Protection), are available for personal and business use.

The simplest way to protect yourself is by using common sense. Take advantage of your provider's security offerings. Protect yourself against viruses. Think twice before using the Net to send really sensitive information. And practice good password control. Never give out your password; keep it unrecognizable (don't use your dog's name or your license tag number), and, if possible, mix numerals, punctuation, and alphabetic characters to make it harder to crack. If you have more than one online account, use a different password for each one.

# Healthy Menus

gopher://gopher.uiuc.edu/Campus Info/Campus Services/Health Services/Health Information/Nutrition

The University of Illinois at Urbana-Champaign (UIUC) Gopher, home to great health and fitness information, is also an excellent resource for food and nutrition topics. Menus focus on eating disorders, weight gain and weight loss, vegetarianism, and healthy diet. Each menu has a selection of relevant, clearly written fact sheets (see Figure 2.12), for example, "Gaining Weight the Healthy Way" and "Eating . . .Healthy Habits, Healthy You." On a related topic, check out "Drinking and Dieting: The Calorie Connection," in the Health Information/Drug_Alcohol menu.

```
Vending Machine Calorie Counter


                    VENDING MACHINE CALORIE COUNTER


FOOD                    Weight            FAT    %CAL
                        (oz.)  CALORIES   (gm.)  FROM FAT
------------------------------------------------------------
CANDY

  Heath Bar             1.3    251        22     79
  Alpine White          1.3    210        14     60
  Mr. Goodbar           1.9    300        20     60
  Skor                  1.4    220        14     57
  Milk Choc. w/Almonds  1.5    230        14     55
  Reese's PB Cup (2)    1.8    280        17     55
  Milk Chocolate Bar    1.7    250        14     50
  Almond Joy            1.8    250        14     50
  Peanut Butter Twix    1.8    260        14     48
  Mounds                1.9    300        16     48
  Whatchamacallit       1.8    260        14     48
  Kit Kat               1.6    250        13     47
  M & M Peanuts         1.7    250        13     47
  M & M Plain           1.7    220        11     45
  Nestle Crunch         2.0    320        16     45
  Snickers              2.1    280        14     45
```

Figure 2.12:
A fact sheet from the UIUC Gopher, "Vending Machine Calorie Counter," presents some eye-opening statistics on favorite snacks from the hallway vending machine.

# FOOD AND NUTRITION BASICS

Nutrition is a complicated topic, especially these days as studies with conflicting results seem to appear regularly. Sometimes you simply want to get basic information: What's in it? Is it safe? How much should I eat? The resources that follow, many sponsored by the U.S. government, offer clearcut and well-documented information with no hype.

# The FDA Almanac

almanac@esusda.gov

The FDA Almanac server was developed to provide an easy and convenient way to access documents on a range of agriculture and food or nutrition-related topics. It specializes in the new food-labeling regulations and provides background information documents on other topics, such as dietary fiber and coronary disease, folic acid and preventing neural tube defects in infants, fruits and vegetables and cancer, and others.

To use the FDA Almanac server, send e-mail to the address above, with the message send fda catalog, to get the list of available files. To receive a user guide, send the message send guide. To order a document, send the message send fda *document-name*. You can request more than one document in each e-mail message, but be sure to place each send command on a separate line. You can search the Almanac with the command search fda *searchterm*. The Almanac server is case sensitive, so type everything in lowercase letters.

# Cornell Cooperative Extension Network

gopher://cce.cornell.edu:70

telnet://empire.cce.cornell.edu

A Cooperative Extension resource, CENET is maintained at the Cornell University Cooperative Extension Service. The Food and Nutrition menu covers timely nutrition topics and food-safety issues. We found an interesting debate over the butter *vs.* margarine issue and research on the wood *vs.* plastic cutting-boards issue. The Mediterranean Diet Pyramid got a thorough going over. Look here too for resources on that traditional Cooperative Extension topic, safe home food preservation. For example, you'll find tips on freezing asparagus.

Other CENET menu choices cover agricultural and environmental topics. You can also reach CENET by Telnet at empire.cce.cornell.edu. Log in as guest (all lowercase); you don't need a password.

## Food Composition Information

gopher://gopher.inforM.umd.edu:70/EdRes/Topic/AgrEnv/USDA

This Gopher site is an alternate route to the USDA Food and Nutrition Information Center (FNIC, see below) and also home to the USDA Food Composition databases. From this site, you can download software—the Dietary Analysis Program—that will analyze your food intake for calories and 27 nutrients and food components. The menu-driven program uses common household measurements and incorporates updated Recommended Dietary Allowances (RDAs) for each nutrient and for 850 foods from the USDA Food Composition database. Along with its other functions, the program effortlessly calculates that mysterious—and important—"percentage of calories from fat" in your diet. Look for the file DAPZ.EXE or DAPZ.ZIP, which is the compressed version.

## Food Safety and Applied Nutrition

http://vm.cfsan.fda.gov:80/list.html

telnet://fdabbs.fda.gov

The Center for Food Safety and Applied Nutrition (CFSAN) is part of the U.S. Food and Drug Administration, and this site combines CFSAN-specific information with links to other FDA information sites and bulletin boards (see Figure 2.13). Look here for consumer advice on food safety, food additives, food contaminants, and similar topics. Sensitive to MSG? Look at the fact sheet here. Another fact sheet discusses the new fat substitutes on the market. For a thorough discussion of common food and drug interactions, get the brochure of the same name from the Consumer Advice link.

Links to other FDA resources include the Bad Bug Book (Foodborne Pathogenic Microorganisms and Natural Toxins) and all FDA regulations. You can search the FDA phone book (and the phone book for the Department of Health and Human Services, for that matter).

The URL for the CFSAN anonymous FTP site is

ftp://anonymous:@vax8.cfsan.fda.gov:21.

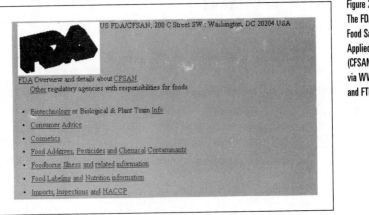

US FDA/CFSAN, 200 C Street SW.; Washington, DC 20204 USA

FDA Overview and details about CFSAN
Other regulatory agencies with responsibilities for foods

- Biotechnology or Biological & Plant Toxin Info
- Consumer Advice
- Cosmetics
- Food Additives, Pesticides and Chemical Contaminants
- Foodborne Illness and related information
- Food Labeling and Nutrition information
- Imports, Inspections and HACCP

**Figure 2.13:**
The FDA's Center for Food Safety and Applied Nutrition (CFSAN) is accessible via WWW, Telnet, and FTP.

## Food and Nutrition Information Center

gopher://cyfer.esusda.gov:70/11/fnic

The Food and Nutrition Information Center (FNIC) Gopher is a service of the National Agricultural Library. Menu choices include the FDA/USDA Food Labeling Information Center, the Food Guide Pyramid, Food Service Management, and Foodborne Illness. You can download publications from the Agriculture Library Forum (ALF) bulletin board menu. Publications include the Nutri-Topics series, lists of peer-reviewed materials "designed to be a starting point for someone looking for information about a specific topic." Nutri-Topics are usually available at consumer, educator, and health-professional levels. Some new titles when we looked were "Nutrition During Pregnancy," "Nutrition and Diabetes," "Nutrition and Cardiovascular Disease," and "Nutrition and Cancer." You'll also find a Gopher link to other resources at the National Agricultural Library.

## Online Personal Nutrition Profile

http://health.mirical.com:80/site/form3.html

What should you be eating? This WWW page presents you with an online questionnaire. Answer the questions about your age, gender, weight, and activity level, and you will receive a personalized analysis of your dietary needs, along with recommended amounts of 29 nutrients from protein, fat, vitamins, and minerals (see Figure 2.14). Completing the questionnaire takes only a few seconds, and you'll receive lots of information.

**On-Line Personal Nutritional Profile**

You can fill out the form below and get back a complete personalized nutritional profile based on the 29 nutrients found in the Personal Food Analyst. Find out the optimum amount of food and nutrients you should be consuming based on your personal attributes.

If you have any questions about how to rate your activity level or other attributes, press the appropriate hot-link below.

**Enter your Personal Information Below**

Name: `Your Name Here`
Age: `34`
Weight: `125` Pounds
Height: `5` ft `5` in
Gender: `Female`        Activity Level `Moderately Active`
Profile: `Norm`

Figure 2.14:
The Mirical On-Line Nutritional Profile page offers a personalized nutrient analysis.

# FOOD AND NUTRITION DISCUSSION LISTS

We all seem to enjoy talking about food almost as much as we enjoy eating it. And when it comes to special nutritional programs or diets, well, we can all use some helpful hints and a little support. On the Internet are a number of discussion lists and newsgroups that deal with food, nutrition, special diets, and weight management. Here's a sampler.

## Very Low-Fat Vegetarian Diet

FATFREE

fatfree-request@hustle.rahul.net

The FATFREE mailing list is well organized and focuses on the practical aspects of eating and cooking for a very low-fat vegetarian diet and on the associated lifestyle issues. The list owner sets the tone right away by sending to all new members a description of the list, guidelines for posting messages, and rules for posting recipes. The clear guidelines seem to help the list avoid the flame wars of some other diet-oriented lists and to help it remain a friendly and helpful spot. Along with the recipes are requests and suggestions for getting the fat out of favorite foods and family recipes, discussions about staying motivated and getting back on the very-low-fat wagon, and specific questions and answers about a whole raft of food and lifestyle issues. FAT-FREE has more than 2000 members, and the message volume is heavy. Get the digest form!

To subscribe, send e-mail to the address above with ADD in the subject line. FATFREE is maintained by a real person, not by a program, so please be polite if you have to wait a bit for a response.

FATFREE recipes are archived at ftp.halcyon.com:/pub/recipes. The list messages are archived (though not forever) at ftp.rahul.net: /pub/artemis/fatfree. You can also get recipes and back issues via e-mail. Send a message to ba-fatfree-request@hustle.rahul.net with the subject archive get help.

## Food and Wine

FOODWINE

listserv@cmuvm.csv.cmich.edu

FOODWINE is an eclectic list that covers almost everything about food or wine or the enjoyment thereof. You'll find good recipes, menu ideas, hints about international foods, and questions and answers on sources for hard-to-find ingredients and products. This list is for people who enjoy food! According to the list owners, "FOODWINE is for serious, but not pedantic, discussion of food, beverages, and related concerns." They liken the list to a "discussion around a *very* large table among people who like to discuss food," and so it is. If you want more than a virtual feast, though, you'll still have to cook it yourself!

> According to the list owners, "FOODWINE is for serious, but not pedantic, discussion of food, beverages, and related concerns."

To subscribe, send e-mail to listserv@cmuvm.csv.cmich.edu with the message SUBSCRIBE FOODWINE Yourfirstname Yourlastname. No subject line is necessary. FOODWINE is archived, so you can mine the "back issues" for recipes or food hints.

# The Vegetarian Lifestyle

VEGLIFE

listserv@vtvm1.cc.vt.edu

VEGLIFE covers a range of topics concerning vegetarian eating, cooking, and lifestyle. If you want to know how to stir-fry tofu or which egg substitutes to use in baking, try this list. VEGLIFE members also discuss lifestyle issues, raising children as vegetarians, for example, although they do so with less heat than members of some other vegetarian discussion lists. The list is international. United Kingdom members report that Burger King there offers vegetarian bean burgers (U.S. members say, "Why not here, BK?"). Europe and Australia also appear well represented.

To subscribe, send e-mail to the address above with the message SUBSCRIBE *Yourfirstname Yourlastname*. No subject line is necessary.

*Don't post commercial messages or advertisements to a mailing list or a newsgroup unless you are specifically invited to do so. Not only is it bad Net manners, it's bad business: You'll alienate far more potential customers than you'll gain.*

# Nutrition and Diet Discussion

sci.med.nutrition

Sci.med.nutrition is an eclectic newsgroup that discusses most things nutritional. You can find talk on the merits of eating breakfast, hints on dietary control of gout, and discourse on just about any vitamin or mineral supplement known to humankind.

# Diets for Weight Loss

DIET

listserv@ubvm.cc.buffalo.edu

DIET is an e-mail discussion list for the support and discussion of weight loss. Freindly, chatty, and amazingly active (sometimes more than 50 messages in one day), DIET seems to fill an important niche in the lives of many of its members, some of whom post several messages a day. Emotional

## Case Matters

On the Internet, whether you type something in upper- or lowercase sometimes matters and sometimes doesn't. Here are a few general guidelines:

- E-mail addresses are not *supposed* to be case-sensitive. Whether you type YourName@address or yourname@address should not make any difference. It's always safer though, and general Internet usage, to type e-mail addresses in all lowercase letters.

- The Unix operating system, which many Internet hosts use, is case sensitive. Unix commands and filenames must be typed exactly as specified. For example, the cd (change directory) command will not work if you type it as CD. Watch your entry of filenames especially. If the directory you're aiming for is /pub/usenet/news.answers, you may never get there if you type Pub/USENET/News.answers.

- Many listserv names are all uppercase, deriving from the BITnet origins of the Listserv program.

- As a matter of good netiquette, never, *never* type your e-mail messages or newsgroup postings in all capital letters. On the Internet, all caps is the equivalent of shouting. Not only is it hard on the eyes, it also suggests anger and invites angry responses. Keep that Caps Lock key turned off!

support is big on this list, for all aspects of life, not just weight management. It's also good for recipe ideas and requests and comments on the role of food in our culture. DIET is generally less political than some of the other diet and nutrition-oriented lists. Be prepared for a full mailbox; better yet, learn to use the Listserv digest option if you sign on to this list!

To subscribe, send e-mail to listserv@ubvm.cc.buffalo.edu with the command SUBSCRIBE DIET *Yourfirstname Yourlastname* in the message. No subject line is needed.

# Accepting Weight Discussion

alt.support.bigfolks

For a totally different take on weight, subscribe to the alt.support.bigfolks newsgroup. This newsgroup supports the acceptance of being fat and is not for the discussion of dieting or surgery for weight loss or weight gain. If you're tired of hearing, reading, and thinking about losing weight, this group may be for you.

Given the recent research, some of it contradictory and controversial, about yo-yo dieting, "fat" genes, and the health effects of obesity, these folks may be onto something.

# Diet Support Group

alt.support.diet

The alt.support.diet newsgroup helps its members through the ups and downs and ins and outs of weight loss and dieting and the associated struggles. In addition to supportive discussions, topics include diet options and discussions of surgery for weight loss, and relevant articles from the national press are posted.

# Obesity Support Group

alt.support.obesity

The alt.support.obesity newsgroup is for people who, generally, are more than 100 pounds overweight and who are trying to lose weight. Discussions include all kinds of topics of interest to people who have a lot of weight to lose, including diets, surgery, pregnancy and obesity, and more.

# RECIPES

If you ever thought the Internet was just for nerdy serious types, think again. Since its beginnings, the Net has served, along with its more serious functions, as a vast, intercontinental recipe exchange. Usenet's traditional recipe and food discussion groups have thrived, and, as the Net has grown, they've branched out to cover particular niche interests. So before you decide what's for dinner, check out some of these recipe resources.

## Recipes Newsgroup

rec.food.recipes

All recipes, all the time. A tasty and quiet corner of the Net with no chatter, no flame wars, just good recipes. Lurk for awhile to see what's cooking, and then post your own recipes to recipes@taronga.com (but read the "Posting Guidelines" file first). A random sampling brought one recipe for Buffalo Wings with half the fat (baked not fried) and another for French Garlic Soup to ward off winter colds.

## Recipe Archives

ftp://anonymous:@ftp.neosoft.com:21/pub/rec.food.recipes

This is the official archive for the rec.food.recipe newsgroup. (see Figure 2.15). A virtual cookbook.

Figure 2.15:
The rec.food.recipes archive starts with this screen and goes on and on!

```
Contents of/pub/rec.food.recipes

Go one level up
    4096 bytes    Apr  9 01:54    appetizers
    2121 bytes    Apr  9 01:54    appetizers-index
    1536 bytes    Mar 27 22:05    barbeque
     623 bytes    Mar 27 22:05    barbeque-index
    4608 bytes    Mar 30 14:50    beans-grains
    2461 bytes    Mar 30 14:49    beans-grains-index
    3584 bytes    Apr  9 01:46    beef-veal
    1966 bytes    Apr  9 01:46    beef-veal-index
    2560 bytes    Mar 28 20:57    beverages
    1321 bytes    Mar 28 20:56    beverages-index
     512 bytes    Mar 26 21:46    breads
    5104 bytes    Apr  9 04:59    breads-index
    6144 bytes    Apr  9 04:30    cakes
    3441 bytes    Apr  9 04:30    cakes-index
    2048 bytes    Mar 28 22:15    candy 945 bytes Mar 28 22:15 candy-ind
```

# Creole and Cajun Cuisine

http://www.webcom.com:80/~gumbo/recipe-page.html

With all this talk about what we should or shouldn't be eating, the dry details of food composition, and the grim realities of food contamination, it's easy to forget that *food is to enjoy*. Not so on the Gumbo pages (see Figure2.16), where Chuck Taggert celebrates the joys of Creole and Cajun cuisine on the Recipe page of the same name and even tries to tell the difference. Be warned, this is not a low-fat recipe site, but if you're ready to *laissez les bon temps roulez*, here's where you can assemble your menu (see Figure 2.17).

> *The Gumbo pages has lots of cultural information links to interesting WWW sites, not to mention cultural information about New Orleans and environs.*

In addition to all the great recipes, the Gumbo pages has lots of cultural information links to interesting WWW sites on food and a culinary tour of recipes from many world and regional cuisines, not to mention cultural information about New Orleans and environs.

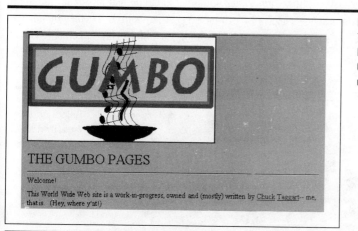

Figure 2.16:
The Gumbo pages are home to wonderful Creole and Cajun recipes.

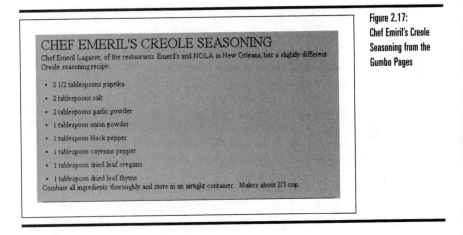

**CHEF EMERIL'S CREOLE SEASONING**

Chef Emeril Lagasse, of the restaurants Emeril's and NOLA in New Orleans, has a slightly different Creole seasoning recipe:

- 2 1/2 tablespoons paprika
- 2 tablespoons salt
- 2 tablespoons garlic powder
- 1 tablespoon onion powder
- 1 tablespoon black pepper
- 1 tablespoon cayenne pepper
- 1 tablespoon dried leaf oregano
- 1 tablespoon dried leaf thyme

Combine all ingredients thoroughly and store in an airtight container. Makes about 2/3 cup.

**Figure 2.17:**
Chef Emiril's Creole Seasoning from the Gumbo Pages

# Veggies Unite!

http://www-sc.ucssc.indiana.edu:80/cgi-bin/recipes/

Veggies Unite! is a searchable archive of more than 1500 vegetarian recipes (see Figure 2.18). Recipes are indexed alphabetically by category. Categories run from Appetizers, Breads, and Casseroles to Sweets, Tofu, and, of course, Veggies. We turned up what's purported to be the real-McCoy Buckingham Palace Scone recipe (for ovo-lactovegetarians only). Whether or not the recipe is authentic, it's good. This WWW site also has links to other food and drink recipe sites and to Internet health, medical, and nutrition sites.

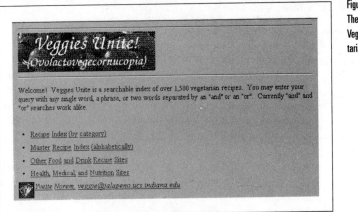

**Figure 2.18:**
The home Page of the Veggies Unite! vegetarian recipe archives

*Veggies Unite!*
*(Ovolactovegecornucopia)*

Welcome! Veggies Unite is a searchable index of over 1,500 vegetarian recipes. You may enter your query with any single word, a phrase, or two words separated by an "and" or an "or". Currently "and" and "or" searches work alike.

- Recipe Index (by category)
- Master Recipe Index (alphabetically)
- Other Food and Drink Recipe Sites
- Health, Medical, and Nutrition Sites

Yvette Norem, veggie@jalapeno.ucs.indiana.edu

# The Electronic Gourmet

http://www.deltanet.com:80/2way/egg/

The electronic Gourmet Guide (eGG) is an Internet e-zine (electronic magazine) devoted to food and recipes (see Figure 2.19). Now a monthly Internet publication, it has the usual magazine features (letters to the editors, columnists, classifieds) plus lots of recipes and links to other WWW resources.

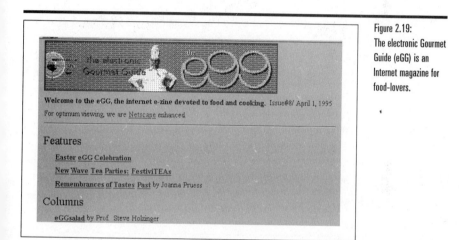

Figure 2.19:
The electronic Gourmet Guide (eGG) is an Internet magazine for food-lovers.

# Coping with Health Challenges

Although a nutritious diet and a fitness program can go a long way toward keeping you healthy, probably nothing can exempt you from facing some of life's health "challenges." None of us is perfect or in perfect health. Whether you have to face the occasional minor illness or deal daily with a chronic condition, you might find yourself in need of some basic health information or some online friends with whom to share your woes.

The first part of this section contains general resources, references, and jumping-off places for finding information about common health problems, minor illnesses, and chronic conditions. The second part contains, in alphabetic order, Internet resources that are concerned with specific problems and conditions.

## THE ONLINE HEALTH-CONCERNS REFERENCE SHELF

Leaf through some of these resources, which are the online equivalent of your family medical guide or favorite health book. All are very sound sources of information on a constellation of health concerns.

## Consumer Health Information

gopher://info.med.yale.edu:70

The Yale Biomedical Gopher is a comprehensive resource that contains some real gems of consumer health information. The Diseases and Disorders menu has documents and connections to resources on AIDS, arthritis, benign prostate disease, diabetes, chronic fatigue syndrome, the flu, and Lyme disease, among others. From here, you can also connect to the Clinical Preventive Services recommendations mentioned earlier in **Part Two** and to dozens of other biomedical Gophers all over the world.

# TJGopher

gopher://tjgopher.tju.edu/11/medical/

Another good place to start a journey through health Gopherspace, the Thomas Jefferson University TJGopher connects you to some of the best health and medical Gophers and other resources around the country. TJGopher itself has resources on AIDS, cancer, diabetes, epilepsy, and more. It also has a version of the Black Bag Medical BBS List and the Handicap BBS list, for those of you ready to venture beyond the Internet into the BBS world.

You can use the TJGopher to reach the cancer resources OncoLink, Cancernet, and the Breast Cancer Information Clearinghouse and to reach the database of genetic diseases (called Online Mendelian Inheritance in Man or *OMIM*) at Johns Hopkins University.

# Clinical Guidelines

gopher://gopher.nlm.nih.gov

The Agency for Health Care Policy and Research (AHCPR) develops clinical guidelines for health-care providers that outline effective treatment plans for a number of conditions. Its goal is "to enhance the quality, appropriateness, and effectiveness of health-care services," and its clinical guidelines have come to represent a standard of care.

The AHCPR Clinical Practice Guidelines cover acute pain management, urinary incontinence, ulcers, cataracts, depression, otitis media in children, benign prostate enlargement, and more. Recommendations generally take the form of clinical practice guidelines for health-care providers and patient-oriented consumer guides.

The Patient's Guide: Pain Control After Surgery, as a good example, is a clearly written guide for patients on how to relieve pain after surgery, covering both drug and nondrug (relaxation, massage, cold packs, TENS [transcutaneous electrical nerve stimulation]) pain-relief strategies. The goal seems to be to put the patient in control and to maximize pain relief, which studies have suggested speeds recovery time and reduces the risks of some postoperative complications.

AHCPR has a guide for parents of children with a particular form of otitis media that helps explain when antibiotic treatment is and isn't warranted (see Figure 2.20).

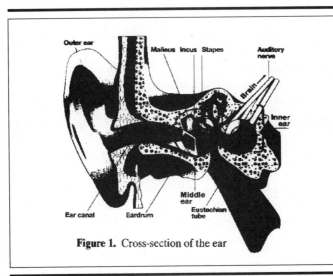

**Figure 2.20:**
Parents of children with ear infections can refer to the AHCPR parents' guide to management of otitis media, which includes this anatomical diagram.

**Figure 1.** Cross-section of the ear

# Privacy?

You can't turn on the news or open a magazine these days without hearing something about computer crime, hackers, privacy issues, or security on the Internet. Before you take the plunge into the Net, you should take a little time to understand the limitations of the medium! After all, nothing as wide open, anarchic, and enormous as the Internet should be assumed to maintain absolute privacy.

With the huge volume of electronic mail on the Internet, the chances that your mail will be read by any one other than the addressee are slim, *but it can happen*. The basic rule of thumb is to put nothing in an e-mail message that you wouldn't put on the back of a postcard. One early Internet admonition was never e-mail anything you wouldn't want to see on the front page of the *New York Times* (or your local paper, for that matter). If you are using your employer's e-mail system, be aware that the privacy of your e-mail is not guaranteed. Recent court cases have supported the right of employers to read employee e-mail.

If you are sending sensitive personal information about your health to an e-mail discussion list or a newsgroup, think carefully about how much you can and should

# Disabilities

gopher://gopher.inform.umd.edu/EdRes/Topic/Disability

The Internet has myriad resources on disabilities. For an excellent starting point, gopher to the University of Maryland and check the Disability Resources menu in inforM Gopher. Along with university, state, and U.S. government information, you'll find information on disability-related e-mail discussion groups and connections to other Gophers and WWW sites.

## ALLERGIES AND ASTHMA

Allergies and asthma are nothing to sneeze at, with millions of sufferers troubled by one or the other. And asthma in children is increasing at an alarming rate. Here are a few Net resources that might be helpful.

reveal in such a public forum. Would your job be compromised if your employer or others found out you have a serious illness? How would you feel if your neighbor finds you in an online discussion of an emotional problem? Maybe you'll feel better (your neighbor's likely there for the same reason you are), but you might not want your personal mental state open to the part of the world that knows you well.

Many e-mail addresses are a recognizable form of a person's name and employer or location. Even if yours is indecipherable, Internet utilities, such as Finger, may translate your user id to your name and system location. Some systems don't allow Finger to get much information about their users; check on yours, or ask your system administrator about the kinds of protections the system offers. Most listserv programs for e-mail can shield your name from the Review feature that lets subscribers view the names of other list members. Send a help message to the listserv address if you need that shield. If you are convinced that you need complete anonymity, check out one of the anonymous mail forwarding systems available on the Net.

## Allergies and Immunology

gopher://lab.allergy.mcg.edu

The Allergy/Immunology Gopher, sponsored by the Medical College of Georgia, is a resource intended for medical professionals and researchers, but some material is relevant for motivated nonprofessionals. The Asthma Online menu cites journal articles, organized by topic, and includes, for example, Acute Asthma, Occupational Asthma, Pharmacotherapy, and Alternative Treatments. If you're willing to tackle the articles in the medical journals, you'll have a shot at doing some of the same reading your health practitioner has been doing.

## Asthma Support Group

alt.support.asthma

The alt.support.asthma newsgroup discusses anything (anything non-commercial, that is) of interest to people who have asthma. Medications, alternative treatments, pets (or coping with other people's pets), and children who have asthma are all popular topics.

## On-line Allergy Center

http://www.sig.net:80/~allergy/welcome.html

The On-line Allergy Center WWW page is produced by an allergist in private practice in Texas. Although much of the material is specific to his practice, this page contains a good short summary of a simple elimination diet for food allergies, some allergy facts (see Figure 2.21) and news, and an article, "Is It a Cold or an Allergy?"

## ARTHRITIS

Arthritis is a disease with many manifestations, some very serious, some chronic and disabling. Arthritis includes more than a hundred conditions, from osteoarthritis to skin problems, such as psoriasis, to autoimmune disorders, such as lupus. The Net has a lot to offer arthritis sufferers in both support and information.

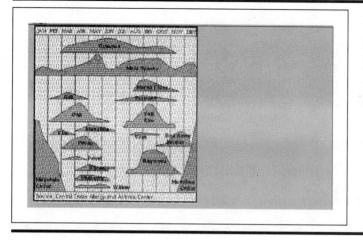

Figure 2.21:
The On-line Allergy Center includes a chart of seasonal allergens (these are from central Texas) over the course of the year.

# Arthritis Foundation Information

ftp://ftp.netcom.com/pub/ar/arthritis/arthritis.html

ftp.netcom.com:/pub/ar/arthritis

The Arthritis Foundation Information Web page (also available via FTP) has an excellent FAQ on arthritis. It also contains ordering information for arthritis-related literature, contact information for the Arthritis Foundation, and a link to the online version of *Arthritis Today* (see Figure 2.22).

# Arthritis Support Groups

alt.support.arhritis

misc.health.arthritis

ARTHRITIS-L

listproc@showme.missouri.edu

These three discussion groups overlap, and members often crosspost, although each group has its loyal followers. In fact, alt.support.arthritis has a "one-way gateway" to ARTHRITIS-L; postings to the newsgroup appear on the mailing list, but mailing list messages do not appear in the newsgroup.

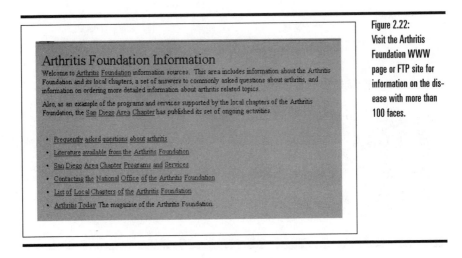

Figure 2.22:
Visit the Arthritis
Foundation WWW
page or FTP site for
information on the dis-
ease with more than
100 faces.

All three discuss the many aspects of arthritis and its many manifestations (more than 100 conditions), from osteoarthritis and rheumatoid
arthritis to psoriasis and gout to auto immune disorders, such as lupus and scle-
roderma. The tone is supportive, and the information exchange ranges from helpful hints to discussions about the latest in drug and alternative therapies. Commercial postings are not permitted.

*The tone is supportive, and the information exchange ranges from helpful hints to in-depth discussions.*

## Arthritis Today

gopher://enews.com/Health and Medical Center/Health & Medical Periodicals

As do all electronic newsstand offerings, Arthritis Today has Table of Contents
listings for back issues, a selection of feature articles, and, of course, subscription information for the hard-copy version. You can download articles
(or e-mail them to yourself). Each issue has an informative arthritis health-
questions-and-answers segment, and we found an interesting article, "Of
Germs and Genes," discussing research on viral and genetic causes of some
forms of arthritis.

# CHRONIC FATIGUE SYNDROME/MYALGIC ENCEPHALOMYELITIS

Chronic fatigue syndrome (CFS) is a condition that has suffered a lot of misunderstanding (including the unfortunate nickname of "yuppie flu") since it first surfaced several years ago. Also known as myalgic encephalomyelitis (primarily in Europe), CFS produces symptoms that include excessive fatigue, general pain, mental fogginess, and often gastrointestinal discomfort.

## Chronic Fatigue Syndrome

http://huizen.dds.nl:80/~cfs-news/

The CFS home page (see Figure 2.23) is less glitzy than many WWW pages, but goes far beyond most in content. You'll find good documents, including the CFS FAQ, information for doctors, a "Dealing with Doctors" primer for CFS patients, information on e-mail and newsgroup discussions, and instructions for network newbies on accessing the CFS electronic resources. From this page you can link to international CFS connections, to resources for related syndromes and conditions, such as Gulf War syndrome, fibromyalgia, fibrositis, Lyme disease, and environmental illness, and of course to other Internet general health resources.

**Figure 2.23:**
The chronic fatigue syndrome home page has a wealth of information on chronic fatigue syndrome and links to resources on related conditions.

Chronic fatigue syndrome / Myalgic encephalomyelitis
Choose category.

- News about CFS/ME

- Information files, and resources for doctors

- Discussion groups

- Other CFS-related pages

- Gateway to the Rest of the World

This web page provided by Roger Burns.
See also the introductory essays about CFS below.

News

- CFS-NEWS Electronic Newsletter-- Latest Edition
- CFS-NEWS Index

# Chronic Fatigue Syndrome Support Group

alt.med.cfs

CFS-L

listserv@list.nih.gov

Chronic fatigue syndrome sufferers took to the Internet early to share stories and support, especially when the condition was less widely known and was considered psychosomatic. The group discusses medical and personal issues and rejoices in sympathetic health providers and sometimes slams those who aren't. Discussions cover medications, aggravating factors, and related

## More . . .

The CFS network users have organized their Internet resources well. For more information, check out these resources from the CFS Index to FAQs. The FTP files can be found at rtfm.mit.edu in directory

> /pub/usenet/news.answers/medicine/chronic-fatigue-syndrome.

◆ Answers to typical questions about chronic fatigue syndrome (CFS FAQ): listserv filename: CFS FAQ (listserv@sjuvm.stjohns.edu), FTP archive name: cfs-faq.

◆ Treatments for chronic fatigue syndrome: listserv filename: CFS TREATMTS (listserv@sjuvm.stjohns.edu), FTP archive name: cfs-treatments.

◆ General resource file for CFS. Lists books, articles, national organizations, newsletters, and electronic discussion groups and files (a large document (60K): Listserv filename: CFS-RES TXT (listserv@sjuvm.stjohns.edu), FTP archive name: cfs-resources.

◆ Computer network resources for CFS on Internet, commercial services, and BBSs. Includes new user advice. Listserv filename: CFS-NET TXT (listserv@sjuvm.stjohns.edu), FTP archive name: cfs-electronic-resources.

◆ For the CFS-NEWS electronic newsletter and CFS Newswire service. Send e-mail to listserv@list.nih.gov with Sub CFS-News *Yourfirst name Yourlastname* in the body of the message. No subject line is needed.

symptoms, and of course lots of emotional support is a primary feature. This group has little sympathy for or interest in commercial postings, no matter how carefully presented.

# DIABETES

Though no longer always the life-threatening illness that it once was, diabetes is still a significant health problem and an illness that requires long-term, often difficult lifestyle changes. The Internet has some excellent diabetes information resources and an active support network.

## Diabetes Discussion

misc.health.diabetes

This newsgroup discusses all aspects of diabetes, including the medical aspects, monitoring, treatments, lifestyle, insurance, social issues, support, and practical concerns. Whether it's discussing the cost of blood glucose monitoring supplies, the pros and cons of insulin pumps, or suitable frostings for wedding cakes, this very active newsgroup has lots of helpful, informative, and supportive input.

For a related group on juvenile diabetes, join alt.support.diabetes.kids, a support group for diabetic children (and their families).

## Diabetes Information

http://www.niddk.nih.gov:80/NIDDK_HomePage.html

The National Institute of Diabetes and Digestive and Kidney Disease (NIDDK) WWW page is a good place to start looking for information on diabetes. Check the section describing the Diabetes Control and Complications Trail and get the e-text pamphlets on Insulin-Dependent Diabetes and diabetic eye disease. Links include the National Institutes of Health (NIH) home page, the National Library of Medicine, and other online health resources from the U.S. government.

## Diabetes Knowledgebase

www.biostat.wisc.edu/diaknow/index.html

Diabetes Knowledgebase, from the University of Wisconsin Medical School, is a treasure trove of resources on diabetes. Start here for easy access to the FAQs from misc.health.diabetes, a great document on online resources for diabetics, and information on groups such as the American Diabetes Association. There's a link to the NIDDK WWW server described above. The Glossary of Diabetes Related Terms is a real gem, with descriptions and definitions in a useful hypertext format (see Figure 2.24).

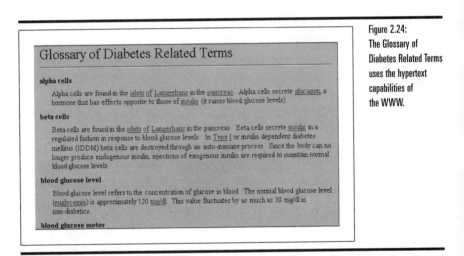

Figure 2.24:
The Glossary of
Diabetes Related Terms
uses the hypertext
capabilities of
the WWW.

## Diabetes Questions and Answers

ftp://rtfm.mit.edu/pub/usenet/news.answers/diabetes/faq/part 1-5

mail-server@rtfm.mit.edu

*message:* send usenet/news.answers/diabetes/faq/part 1-5

The Diabetes FAQ, which is composed of five files, has been compiled from the answers to the questions most frequently asked in the mis.health.diabetes newsgroup. To name only a few examples, it covers blood glucose monitoring, treatments, and research and is loaded with solutions to practical problems.

In addition to the sources noted above for it, the Diabetes FAQ is posted regularly to the misc.health.diabetes newsgroup and is available on WWW at http://www.cis.ohio-state.edu/hypertext/faq/usenet/diabetes/top.html.

*Quote sparingly from the original message when you're responding to e-mail or to a newsgroup posting. No one wants to read the original message again and again, especially if he or she has expensive, long-distance phone access to the Internet. Keep your messages, your subject line, and your .sig files short and to the point.*

## DIGESTIVE AILMENTS

Few of us get through life without dealing at some point with minor digestive ailments; some of us have to deal with chronic digestive problems. Either way, you can find some excellent information on the Internet and some good support if you have long-term problems.

## Crohn's Disease and Ulcerative Colitis

http://qurlyjoe.bu.edu:80/cduchome.html

The Crohn's Disease/Ulcerative Colitis home page is a good basic source for information on these conditions. Look for FAQs on irritable bowel syndrome, inflammatory bowel disease, and collagenous colitis. This WWW page has its roots in the alt.support.crohns-colitis newsgroup, so of course it contains a link to that newsgroup and to the alt.support.ostomy newsgroup as well.

## Information on Digestive Problems

http://www.niddk.nih.gov:80/NIDDK_HomePage.html

The National Institute of Diabetes and Digestive and Kidney Disease (NIDDK) home page mentioned above is a must visit for people with digestive problems. Look for the documents on heartburn, and hiatal hernia (officially, Gastroesophogeal Reflux Disease, or GERD), and lactose intolerance.

# LOW BACK PAIN

Back injury and associated low back pain is one of the leading causes of time lost from work due to disability. Treatments for back problems have changed considerably over the last decade or so. The Internet has some interesting resources for back pain sufferers.

## Back Pain

salus.med.uvm.edu:70/1/HEALTH CARE AND MEDICAL INFORMATION/Diseases and Disorders/Back Pain

This Back Pain Gopher menu is from the University of Vermont (also home to the Vermont Rehabilitation Engineering Research Center, which has the only U.S. government research grant on back pain and the Backs-L e-mail discussion list). On this Gopher are documents and resources for preventing and coping with back pain, especially occupation-related back pain.

## Back Pain Research

BACKS-L

listproc@moose.uvm.edu

The BACKS-L discussion list is for those researching back pain causes and treatments, but if you're troubled with back problems, it can be a good place to lurk. The list owner discourages personal requests for clinical information but does allow requests for feedback on specific devices and treatments. BACKS-L is a low-volume list

To subscribe, send e-mail to the address above with the message Subscribe BACKS-L *Yourfirstname Yourlastname.* No subject line is needed.

# MEDICATIONS AND TESTS

It's up to you, as a good health consumer, to inform yourself about the medications and diagnostic procedures your physician orders for you. No doubt your physician will fill you in, as will pharmacists and technicians, but here are some Internet resources for further research.

# Food and Drug Administration Bulletin Board System

telnet://telnet fdabbs.fda.gov

The Food and Drug Administration (FDA) bulletin board system is a good source for up-to-date information on newly approved drugs and medical devices and carries news information from the FDA. You'll find an index to the *FDA Consumer* magazine and selected articles, drug bulletins, and AIDS information.

The login for the FDA BBS system is bbs. For a list of available commands, type help. For a list of topics, type topics; to log off, type quit.

# Home Tests

http://kerouac.pharm.uky.edu:80/KitsHP.html

From the University of Kentucky College of Pharmacy, this home page (see Figure 2.25) gives the low-down on equipment for monitoring high blood pressure and blood glucose at home and for do-it-yourself kits for testing for pregnancy, predicting ovulation, and screening for colorectal cancer. There is a definite retail pharmacist slant here, giving the kind of information a pharmacist might need to decide which merchandise to carry and how to advise and instruct the customer/patient on purchase and use.

---

Home Test Kits Homepage

Table of Contents

Blood Pressure Monitors

Colorectal Cancer Home Testing Kits

Glucose Monitoring Kits

Ovulation Prediction Kits

Pregnancy Home Testing Kits

Return to Collge of Pharmacy Homepage

Questions and comments, please write to Amanda Tatro,

**Figure 2.25:**
The Home Test Kits Homepage from the University of Kentucky School of Pharmacy has information on common home screening tests and monitoring equipment.

## Pharmaceutical Information

http://pharminfo.com/

The Pharmaceutical Information Network is a commercial Internet site that provides pharmaceutical information to pharmacists, physicians, and patients (see Figure 2.26). You'll find technical articles on specific drugs taken from the page sponsor's publications, Frequently Asked Questions about drugs (with responses), a commercial area for pharmaceutical-related businesses, and an archive of the sci.med.pharmacy newsgroups. Links to other Internet pharmacy sites round out the page. Most articles are technical and would be of interest only if you've been prescribed a specific drug, but some, "America's 80 Billion Aspirin Habit," for example, are of more general interest.

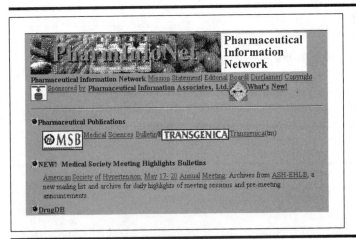

Figure 2.26:
The Pharmaceutical Information Network is a source for technical and general interest information on prescription and over-the-counter drugs.

## Tests and Procedures

gopher.uiuc.edu/UI/CSF/health/heainfo/test

The University of Illinois McKinley Health Center Gopher rewards us with clear descriptions of 11 common diagnostic tests and procedures (from barium enema to upper GI series). The fact sheets outline test procedures, pretest requirements, and causes of false negative and false positive results and give you an idea of how you might feel during the procedure. If you think one of these procedures might be in your future, read here first. If you're scheduled for one of the tests described, your own health-care provider's instructions should of course take precedence over information from this Gopher.

# MIGRAINE HEADACHES

More than 23 million Americans suffer from migraine headaches, which can range from being inconvenient at best to severely debilitating at their worst. Migraine sufferers have come to use the Net as a means to support one another and to share information on new treatments.

## Migraine Questions and Answers

ftp://julian.uwo.ca/doc/FAQ/alt.support.headaches.migraine

The Migraine FAQ is a succinct and thorough discussion of the types of migraines, symptoms, causes, triggers, and treatments. The current drugs (and their side effects) for migraine are listed. The FAQ includes a bibliography of book resources, contact information for helpful associations and headache clinics, and equipment sources.

## Migraine Support Group

alt.support.headaches.migraine

The alt.support.headaches.migraine newsgroup gives at least some migraine sufferers a place to share information, experiences, and coping strategies. According to the newsgroup's charter, the discussion is open to "anyone who wishes to state their experiences and share the knowledge of dealing and living with chronic head pain." Discussions cover drug and nondrug treatments, migraine triggers, and general support.

# MINOR AILMENTS

Sometimes minor, common illnesses cause us as much concern as more serious problems. After all, we're more likely to try to manage minor ailments on our own; none of us wants to run to our health-care provider with every sniffle. Here are some good sources to help you get information on more common problems.

## Common Illnesses Healthline

gopher://healthline.umt.edu:700/General Health Information

Healthline from the University of Montana is another of the standby general-interest health resources. Healthline has some good material for coping with minor or chronic illness. Look here for clearly written, informative patient fact sheets on the common cold, stomach flu, asthma, cystitis, "pinkeye" (conjunctivitis), mononucleosis, hay fever, back pain, and headaches.

## Consumer Health Information

gopher://gopher.health.state.ny.us:70

The New York State Department of Health sponsors this Gopher, which focuses on consumer health information of both general and state-specific interest. The Communicable Diseases menu has fact sheets on 59 communicable diseases, from amebiasis to yersinosis, as well as fact sheets on more common concerns, such as influenza, measles, and swimmer's itch (see Figure 2.27).

```
NEW YORK STATE DEPARTMENT OF HEALTH
|
Fifth Disease              (erythema infectiosum, parvovirus B19 infection

What is fifth disease?

Fifth disease is a viral infection which often affects red blood cells. It
is caused by a human parvovirus (B19). For many years, fifth disease was
viewed as an unimportant rash illness of children. Recently, studies have
shown that the virus may be responsible for serious complications in certain
individuals.

Who gets fifth disease?

Anyone can be infected, but the disease seems to occur more often in
elementary school-age children.

How is the virus spread?

The virus is spread by exposure to airborne droplets from the nose and throa
of infected people.

What are the symptoms and when do they appear?

One to two weeks after exposure, some children will experience a low grade
fever and tiredness. By the third week, a red rash generally appears on the
cheeks giving a slapped face appearance. The rash may then extend to the bod
```

**Figure 2.27:**
The New York State Department of Health Gopher has fact sheets on communicable diseases, including this one on Fifth Disease, a common minor childhood illness that may occasionally be responsible for serious complications.

The Environmental and Occupational Health menu has a guide to reference materials on toxic substances, an introduction to toxic substances, a glossary of environmental health terms, and a description of a power lines project on electric and magnetic fields. Consumer guides describe home-care services and how to find a nursing home.

## Health Information, University of Illinois at Urbana-Champaign

gopher://gopher.uiuc.edu/UI/CSF/health/heainfo/

The University of Illinois at Urbana-Champaign McKinley Health Center Gopher is a great source for well-prepared documents on common health problems. Look in the Diseases/Conditions menu for information on asthma, blood pressure, the common cold, headaches, even warts. Check the Contagious/Communicable Diseases submenu for head lice, hepatitis, and mumps, and check the Miscellaneous submenu for acne, cerumen (ear wax), frostbite, and ear infections.

## REPETITIVE STRAIN INJURY/CARPAL TUNNEL SYNDROME

Repetitive strain injury (RSI) and carpal tunnel syndrome (CTS) are conditions brought about by constant trauma to the affected area, usually the results of poor working habits or conditions. The two conditions (CTS is a type of repetitive strain injury) constitute the fastest growing category of work-related disability. Because so many computer users have been at risk, the Internet has been particularly helpful to RSI/CTS sufferers who want to share information and give and receive support.

## Carpal Tunnel Syndrome

http://www.cyberport.net:80/mmg/cts/ctsintro.html

This Web page is a sample of a commercial patient education product, but even so it has some excellent information and great graphics on carpal tunnel syndrome. The text information covers anatomy and physiology and the diagnosis and treatment of carpal tunnel syndrome (see Figure 2.28). Information about the company is included on the home page.

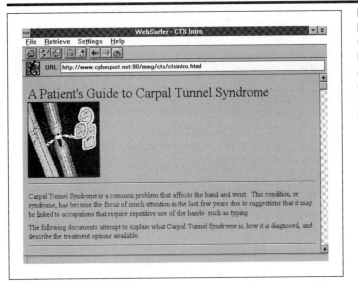

Figure 2.28:
If you wonder why your hands and wrists hurt after hours at the computer keyboard, check out the Carpal Tunnel Syndrome Introduction page.

# Carpal Tunnel Syndrome Discussion

SOREHAND

sorehand@uscsfvm.bitnet

The SOREHAND discussion group talks about any and all topics concerning carpal tunnel syndrome, repetitive strain injury, and related conditions. Because this condition is often derived from and affects people's work, employer support (or the lack of it) is a big topic. Discussions of diagnoses and treatments are common, as are searches for understanding health-care providers. Other hot topics are coping strategies and assistive technology (not surprisingly, most of the list members work on—and owe their injuries to—computers), such as dictation software. SOREHAND is a busy list. Get the digest form.

To subscribe, send e-mail to the address above with the message Subscribe SOREHAND *Yourfirstname Yourlastname*. No subject line is necessary.

*Never post other people's private e-mail to a mailing list or a newsgroup. It's a serious violation of privacy and a very big netiquette faux pas.*

## Repetitive Strain Injury

RSI

majordomo@world.std.com

This regularly published newsletter is produced for and by sufferers of repetitive stress injury and carpal tunnel syndrome. To subscribe, send e-mail to the address above with the one word message Subscribe. No subject line or name is needed.

## SLEEP

Do you have trouble falling sleep, staying asleep, sleeping when you shouldn't, or snoring and snorting through the night? Sleep disorders cause accidents and lost productivity and disrupt families and personal lives. And they are far more common—and more serious—than you might imagine. Visit these Internet resources to learn more.

## Sleep Apnea Questions and Answers

http://www.access.digex.net:80/~faust/sldord/osa/osa.faq.html

The basics about Sleep Apnea (or Apnoea, as it's spelled in this FAQ) were written by someone who has experienced it. Symptoms are clearly described ("How do I know if I have it?"), and the available treatments are discussed from a patient's perspective.

## Sleep Disorders Support Group

alt.support.sleep-disorders

This group provides support and practical suggestions for those with sleep disorders. Posters to this group seem to run the gamut of sleep disorder manifestations. Discussions concern diagnoses and treatments, finding a sleep disorders clinic, and support issues.

## Sleep Medicine

http://www.cloud9.net/~thorpy/

Visit this WWW resource for helpful information on all kinds of sleep disorders. The Sleep Medicine home page (see Figure 2.29) is a resource for health-care workers and consumers alike. It contains excellent information on sleep apnea, a dangerous condition that often masquerades as snoring, children's sleep problems (including bedwetting), narcolepsy (falling asleep at inappropriate times), and lots more. If you're having trouble falling asleep, try the document "Dos and Don'ts for Poor Sleepers," and for some historical perspective, see "On Sleep and Sleeplessness" (Aristotle, 350 BC).

The Sleep Medicine home page will point you to online support groups, sleep disorder clinics, professional and patient organizations, books and periodicals, and more. There are FTP and WWW links to the Australian National SIDS (Sudden Infant Death Syndrome) database and clinical guidelines for infant sleep apnea, believed to cause some SIDS deaths.

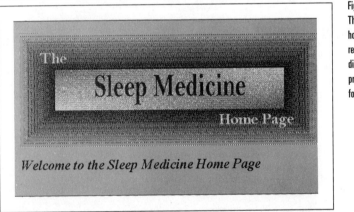

**Figure 2.29:**
The Sleep Medicine home page has resources on sleep disorders for health professionals and for patients.

# Facing Serious Illness

We're never more alone than when we face a serious illness, and yet there are few times in life when we need the help of other people more. Not only does a serious illness present physical challenges of pain and distress, but it's frightening. We are often plunged into a world where we don't understand the vocabulary or the Byzantine ways of the health-care system.

The Internet's health resources can be a real life-support system for people—either patients or their families—facing serious illness. You can use the Internet to seek out the latest information on the illness, read patient education materials and medical reports, learn about medications and treatments, and locate specialty clinics and experts. You can seek emotional support and exchange information and coping strategies in the newsgroups and mailing lists with people who have already made it through the struggles you're facing and with those who, like you, are just beginning the journey.

> *The Internet's health resources can be a real life-support system for people—either patients or their families—facing serious illness.*

Internet resources for serious illnesses vary a great deal in tone, approach, and content. Some are aimed directly at patients and are easy to understand; others are professional medical resources and may, if you're not prepared, be incomprehensible or even intimidating. Much more information is available about some diseases, for example, cancer, than others, but whatever illness you face, you can probably find useful information on the Net if you persist in your search.

The first part of this section contains general resources, references, and jumping-off places for finding information about a range of diseases and conditions. The second part contains Internet resources for some all-too-common serious health problems and conditions.

## THE ONLINE SERIOUS-ILLNESS REFERENCE SHELF

The academic medical community has been discovering the Internet in a big way, and as a result, a number of medical schools and major medical centers have devoted some significant resources to getting information up on the Net. That's good news if you need health information on more serious conditions or of a more technical nature. Here are some good general medical resources with which to start an Internet search.

### The Virtual Hospital™

http://vh.radiology.uiowa.edu:80

The Virtual Hospital (see Figure 2.30) presented by the University of Iowa College of Medicine is a great example of how the Web can be used in medicine and medical education. Most resources in the Virtual Hospital are targeted at medical professionals and medical students, but there is some excellent patient-oriented material as well. And if you have a serious illness, you're probably educating yourself on your disease and learning the appropriate medical vocabulary. So browse the departments of the Virtual Hospital to see what might be of use to you. The Virtual Hospital is a true multimedia resource, stocked with audio and images.

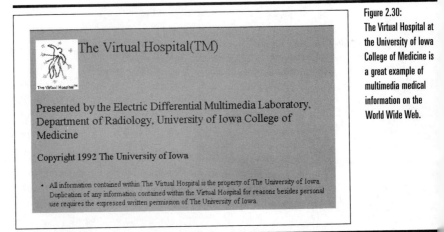

The Virtual Hospital(TM)

Presented by the Electric Differential Multimedia Laboratory, Department of Radiology, University of Iowa College of Medicine

Copyright 1992 The University of Iowa

• All information contained within The Virtual Hospital is the property of The University of Iowa. Duplication of any information contained within the Virtual Hospital for reasons besides personal use requires the expressed written permission of The University of Iowa.

Figure 2.30:
The Virtual Hospital at the University of Iowa College of Medicine is a great example of multimedia medical information on the World Wide Web.

# Medical Specialty Information

http://galaxy.einet.net

If you're in need of resources on serious illnesses, you'll want to go to yet another central Web site, Galaxy (see Figure 2.31), which has an excellent selection of links to medical specialty information. From the index, choose the Medicine entry and then choose Medical Specialties. Galaxy also has some wonderful search capabilities to help you find information on specific topics.

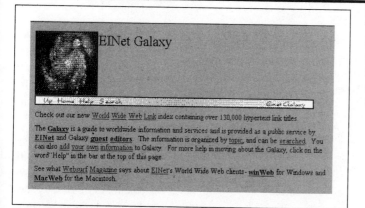

**Figure 2.31:**
The Galaxy home page has excellent WWW search facilities and information on medicine and medical specialties.

# Med Help Medical Information

http://medhlp.netusa.net/

telnet://telnet medhlp.netusa.net

ftp://ftp medhlp.netusa.net

Med Help International (see Figure 2.32) provides medical information, in nontechnical terminology, on a range of topics. As are many Internet

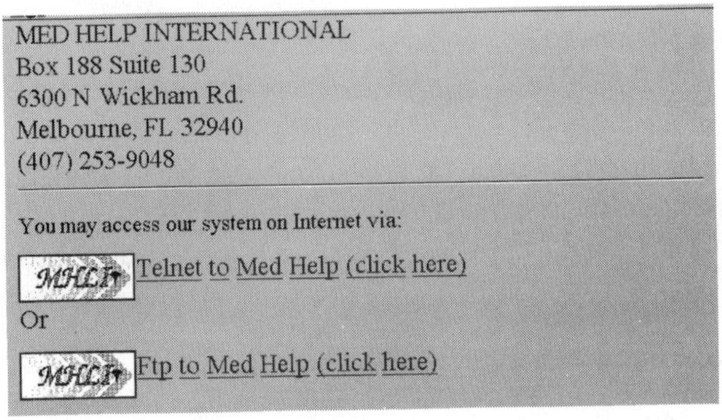

MED HELP INTERNATIONAL
Box 188 Suite 130
6300 N Wickham Rd.
Melbourne, FL 32940
(407) 253-9048

You may access our system on Internet via:

*MHLI* Telnet to Med Help (click here)
Or

*MHLI* Ftp to Med Help (click here)

Figure 2.32:
Med Help has a WWW
interface for its Telnet
and FTP connections.

resources, Med Help is a volunteer endeavor, organized by two people who needed access to similar information at a time of serious family illness. It is staffed by volunteer physicians and health professionals.

Med Help has 12 "libraries," including those devoted to information on brain tumors, cancer, and related topics and those for National Cancer Institute patient information, diseases, drugs and pharmaceuticals, medical news and bulletins, and women's health issues (see Figure 2.33). Each "library" contains documents—always in lay person's terminology—on specific topics in its category.

*The Diseases Library, for example, contains more than 150 documents on topics from aging and hearing loss to myasthenia gravis to retinitis pigmentosa to Wolff Parkinson White syndrome.*

Resources cover common and uncommon conditions and minor and serious illnesses. The Diseases Library, for example, contains more than 150 documents on topics from aging and hearing loss to myasthenia gravis to retinitis pigmentosa to Wolff Parkinson White syndrome. Documents often cite sources for further reading and provide information about who to contact for more information or for support.

Figure 2.33:
The Med Help libraries
index

```
:Your current Library selected is:
:NEWS    -News/Bulletins & Long Lived Information    UQ8 3   :   :
:                                                    333 CD? : 3   :
HHHHHHHHHHHHHHHHHHHHHHHHHHHHHHHHHHHHHHHHHHHHHHHHHHHHHHHHHHHHHHHHHH<
   Please select one of the above items    s

Select a Library (or '?' for a list): ?

  Library   Files  Description
  -------   -----  ------------------------------------------------
  BRAINTMR     20  Brain tumor library
  CANCER      148  Cancer and Related Information
  CANCER2     105  National Cancer Inst. Patient Info Files
  DISEASES    220  Diseases of the human body
  DRUGS        22  Drug/Pharmacutical information
  MAIN         13  General Med Help Information
  NEWS         49  News/Bulletins & Long Lived Information
  PROCS         7  Medical Procedures and Tests
  SOFTWARE     30  Shareware and Freeware Programs
  SUPPORT      33  Support Groups and Medical Support Info
  UPLOAD      DOS  User Uploads to Med Help
  W-HEALTH     17  Women's Health Issues

Select a Library (or '?' for a list): █
```

Look at the News Library for updates on medical topics and at the Drugs Library for information on new and experimental drugs. Med Help also tries to serve as "a 'clearing house' for patient support groups, in an effort to have all the various groups represented in one place." The staff will also do searches on specific topics for a reasonable fee.

Med Help's Web address was solely a connection to its Telnet and FTP servers when we visited. The Telnet application is menu based and relatively easy to use. Log in as new, and the program will take you through some introductory sign-in procedures. Med Help also has forums, e-mail, and teleconferences to facilitate communication among its users.

# AIDS

Because AIDS has had a global impact, the Internet was a natural venue for sharing research information, epidemiological data, and treatment and prevention strategies. It has also been the vehicle for the development of an international support network for AIDS patients and advocates.

# AIDS Information

http://www.actwin.com:80/aids/vl.html

The WWW Virtual Library on AIDS is a collection of links to major AIDS-related resources, including the <u>World Health Organization Global Programme on AIDS</u> (and full text of all its AIDS publications), the <u>National Library of Medicine</u>, <u>National Institutes of Health</u>, <u>Cyberzine's AIDS Information</u>, and many, many more. This is a good place to start looking around for AIDS information (see Figure 2.34).

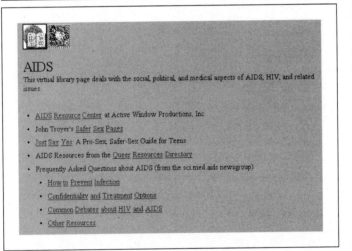

**Figure 2.34:**
The WWW Virtual Library on AIDS is an excellent place to start a search of the Internet for AIDS-related information.

# AIDS Medical/Scientific Discussion

sci.med.aids

The sci.med.aids newsgroup is an excellent example of the important function newsgroups can play in health-related fields. This is a *medical* discussion with regular postings of the CDC Daily Summaries and the VA AIDS Information Newsletter. Lots of good information on AIDS, HIV, ARC, treatments, prevention, and more.

## AIDS Questions and Answers

ftp://rtfm.mit.edu/pub/usenet/news.answers/aids-faq

http://www.cis.ohio-state.edu:80/hypertext/faq/usenet

gopher://family.hampshire.edu/Reproductive Medical and Health Issues/sci.med.aids Frequently Asked Questions.

The sci.med.aids FAQ is posted regularly to sci.med.aids, misc.health.aids, and several other newsgroups. You can also FTP the document (it comes in several parts, so be sure to get them all) from rtfm.mit.edu and access it via the WWW and 'Gopher.

## HIVNET

gopher://gopher.hivnet.org

HIVNET is an international AIDS resource, based in Europe, that contains a wealth of documents on all aspects of AIDS/HIV prevention and treatment in several languages, from Afrikaans to Russian. The Gopher has connections to other AIDS-related Gophers and to an extensive list of AIDS-related magazines and journals, including, for example, searchable archives of *AIDS Treatment News*. HIVNET also runs an e-mail server (send the e-mail message SEND HELP to mail-server@hivnet.org).

For WWW access, go to http://www.hivnet.org, and for FTP access, go to ftp://ftp.hivnet.org.

## Global AIDS and HIV Resources

http://www.ircam.fr:80/solidarites/sida/index-e.html

This French Web site (see Figure 2.35) has excellent links (in English and in French) to global AIDS information. The site has information on counseling and support and links to databases, publications, prevention information, nursing and AIDS, and conventional and alternative treatments.

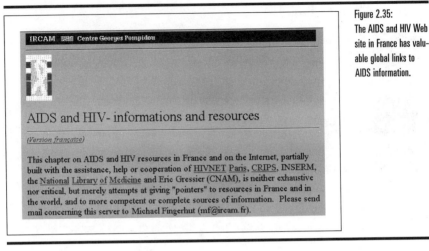

Figure 2.35:
The AIDS and HIV Web site in France has valuable global links to AIDS information.

## U.S. Government AIDS Information

gopher://odie.niaid.nih.gov

The National Institute for Allergy and Infectious Diseases (NIAID) AIDS Gopher is a premier resource for AIDS information and connections to other AIDS resources. Stop here first for information on AIDS studies and for connections to all the other U.S. government resources on AIDS, including the Centers for Disease Control and the National Commission on AIDS. In addition, you will find here a searchable glossary of AIDS terminology, dozens of downloadable documents and articles, and NIAID pamphlets on sexually transmitted diseases.

## AIDS Daily Summary

gopher://gopher.niaid.nih.gov:70

The Centers for Disease Control publishes this daily clipping service with articles about HIV/AIDS in the press and in medical journals. Perusing the AIDS Daily Summary is a great way to stay on top of new developments.

# VA AIDS Information

gopher.niaid.nih.gov:70

This electronic newsletter is a longer and more medically oriented biweekly from the U.S. Department of Veterans Affairs AIDS Information Center in San Francisco. It is also posted on some newsgroups and is available via many Gopher connections.

## ALZHEIMER'S DISEASE

Look for Internet resources on Alzheimer's disease that not only educate and enlighten on the condition itself, but also attempt to lighten the load on the family members and caregivers of Alzheimer's sufferers.

# Alzheimer Resources

http://werple.mira.net.au/~dhs/ad.html

The Alzheimer Web home page is a resource on Alzheimer's disease for researchers and for patients and their families. The site has a collection of documents and links that would be helpful to anyone dealing with the disease.

Look for answers to common questions about the disease, a selection of articles, and a bibliography of recommended books (most fairly technical). A real gem is an ASCII database of important scientific papers on Alzheimer's that you can download and, if you want, search using simple word-processor search functions. There's even a case study of the Magnetic Resonance Imaging (MRI) of an Alzheimer's patient brain (see Figure 2.36), complete with video (which you can look at if your Web browser has an MPEG viewer).

You can also find a list of researchers working on Alzheimer's disease and a directory of research labs and their home pages.

Links to other Internet sites and a Lycos Web search facility round out this excellent resource.

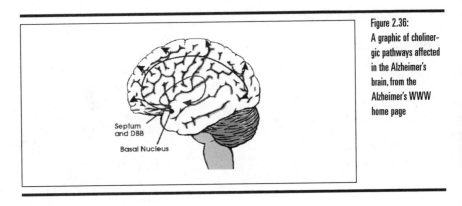

Figure 2.36:
A graphic of choliner-
gic pathways affected
in the Alzheimer's
brain, from the
Alzheimer's WWW
home page

Septum
and DBB

Basal Nucleus

## Alzheimer's and Dementia

http://teri.bio.uci.edu

Another Alzheimer's home page, this one from the University of California at
Irvine, has glitzy graphics and information on diagnostic imaging, on
research, and on dementia. Check out the Frequently Asked Questions section and the glossary.

### Cyberspace and the (Lost) Art of Letter-Writing

It's been said that the art of letter-writing, thought to be on the wane since the
advent of the telephone, is going to be revitalized in cyberspace in the form of
elegant and eloquent electronic mail letters and newsgroup postings.

We may be near the dawn of a new millennium in written communication, but
the state of our discourse on the Net indicates that we're not there quite yet. Yes,
some Net denizens write perfect Net prose, but most of the rest of us are either too
wordy or too terse, too pedantic or too slangy. And far too many of us seem to have
left our spell-checkers and grammar software—and our manners sometimes—
back at the gates of the Internet.

So here, Gentle Readers, are a few guidelines for more felicitous Net prose and
more effective communications overall:

◆   In the interest of conserving bandwidth *and* making the most of the
     medium, we should strive for "Goldilocks-size" postings that are neither

# Alzheimer Discussion

ALZHEIMER

majordomo@wubios.wustl.ed

ALZHEIMER is an e-mail discussion group for patients and their families, caregivers, and others. To subscribe, send email to the address above with the message subscribe ALZHEIMER. No subject line or name is necessary.

## CANCER

The Net has a wealth of resources on cancer, and excellent resources at that. From the CANCERNET documents provided by the National Cancer Institute to the wide-ranging and compassionate online cancer support groups, the Internet can make a big difference in the lives of people with cancer—and in the lives of their families.

too long nor too short, but just right for what we have to say. Rereading Strunk and White's *Elements of Style* might do us all some good.

♦ If we let our spelling and grammar lapse because we're in a hurry, we risk diminishing the impact of our message (in the eyes of some at least) and distracting our readers.

♦ IMHO (In My Humble Opinion), we should let abbreviations such as that one become a distinguished part of Net history and lore. Almost every sentence, BTW (By The Way), could stand perfectly well without them (Are you beginning to see what I mean?); and half the people can't decipher them half the time anyway.

♦ Let's keep in mind that the purpose of sending these messages into cyberspace is to *communicate* with the real human beings on the other end. Clarity and courtesy ought to be our watchwords.

## Cansearch

http://www.access.digex.net/~mkragen/cansearch.html

If the Internet had road signs, Cansearch would likely have one that read "Start Here for Cancer Information." Cansearch is the home page of the National Coalition for Cancer Survivorship, which Marshall Kragen developed and maintains. Cansearch is an excellent place to begin a search for Internet resources on cancer. Using Cansearch, cancer patients and their families can find information and support as they deal with the medical, emotional, and spiritual impacts of the disease (see Figure 2.37).

> *Cansearch is an excellent place to begin a search for Internet resources on cancer.*

Kragen takes his readers by the hand and gently leads them through the maze of Internet cancer resources, suggesting where to go first, how to use a given resource, and where to find more information.

Links to other resources include <u>CANCERNET</u>, <u>OncoLink</u>, <u>Cancer News</u>, <u>Clinical Trials</u>, the <u>National Cancer Institute</u>, and lots more. There are also pointers to the online support groups for cancer patients and their families.

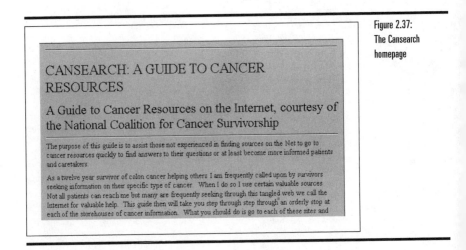

Figure 2.37:
The Cansearch
homepage

CANSEARCH: A GUIDE TO CANCER RESOURCES

A Guide to Cancer Resources on the Internet, courtesy of the National Coalition for Cancer Survivorship

The purpose of this guide is to assist those not experienced in finding sources on the Net to go to cancer resources quickly to find answers to their questions or at least become more informed patients and caretakers.

As a twelve year survivor of colon cancer helping others I am frequently called upon by survivors seeking information on their specific type of cancer. When I do so I use certain valuable sources. Not all patients can reach me but many are frequently seeking through this tangled web we call the Internet for valuable help. This guide then will take you step through step through an orderly stop at each of the storehouses of cancer information. What you should do is go to each of these sites and

## Cancer Questions and Answers

gopher://nysernet.org/

The Cancer FAQ is posted in a number of spots, including this one at the Breast Cancer Information Clearinghouse on the NYSERNet Gopher. It is an excellent resource for tracking down Internet and other online cancer resources.

## Cancer Discussion

CANCER-L

listserv@wvnvm.bitnet

If Cansearch is the place to begin an information search on cancer, CANCER-L is the place to seek support and fellow travelers. CANCER-L probably epitomizes the best of the Internet when it comes to online support and information sharing. CANCER-L is for cancer patients, survivors, and their families and is an unexcelled source of emotional support and information exchange. The list participants are compassionate and kind (flame wars seem pretty out of place here) and quick to welcome new members. List members follow one another's progress, rejoice at good test results, and share sorrow when the news isn't as positive. Practical tips and clinical information are also shared.

> *CANCER-L probably epitomizes the best of the Internet when it comes to online support and information sharing.*

*Avoid crossposting the same message to different groups. Unless it's an informational resource (and never a commercial or an advertising message) that needs widespread distribution, it's best to post to one forum only. Many people subscribe to related lists or newsgroups, and it's not a good use of bandwidth for them to get umpteen copies of your post (not to mention that it can be pretty irritating to read the same message several times). If your message has wide appeal, interested readers will see that it does get reposted to other groups and/or lists.*

## CANCERNET Data

cancernet@icicb.nci.nih.gov

http://www.nih.gov

CANCERNET is a great example of your government at work for you online. Using e-mail, you can request cancer information from the National Cancer Institute (NCI) in the form of information statements from the NCI's Physician Data Query (PDQ) database, fact sheets on various cancer topics from the NCI's Office of Cancer Communications, and citations and abstracts on selected topics from the CANCERLIT database. Some information is also available in Spanish.

To receive a list of available documents and instructions, send e-mail to the address above, with the message help. If you have the contents list and want to order a document, enter the item's code from the contents list (see Figure 2.38). For more than one document, enter the code for each on a separate line in the e-mail message. Use the same address.

CANCERNET is also available on a number of Gophers. For an up-to-date listing of all the Gopher sites, e-mail the above address to request item cn-400030 from CANCERNET.

```
Date:     Thu, 20 Apr 1995 00:18:27
From:     cancernet-request@icicb.nci.ni    To: jcryer@mv.MV.COM
Subject:  Your response from CANCERNE

CANCER SCREENING AND PREVENTION
Overview
   Cancer Prevention. . . . . . . . . . . . cn-304750
   Cancer Screening . . . . . . . . . . . . cn-303092
Aerodigestive Tract Cancer (head & neck, esophagus, lung)
   Prevention. . . . . . . . . . . . . . . . cn-305233
Breast Cancer
   Screening . . . . . . . . . . . . . . . . cn-304723
Cervical Cancer
   Prevention. . . . . . . . . . . . . . . . cn-304734
   Screening . . . . . . . . . . . . . . . . cn-304728
Colorectal Cancer
   Prevention. . . . . . . . . . . . . . . . cn-304731
   Screening . . . . . . . . . . . . . . . . cn-304726
Gastric (Stomach) Cancer
   Screening . . . . . . . . . . . . . . . . cn-304880
```

Figure 2.38: These PDQ Cancer Screening and Prevention Summaries are only one screenful of the many cancer fact sheets and documents available via e-mail from CANCERNET.

# OncoLink

http://cancer.med.upenn.edu

OncoLink (see Figure 2.39), from the University of Pennsylvania Medical School, is a premier reference for information on all aspects of cancer: clinical, physical, emotional, spiritual, and financial.

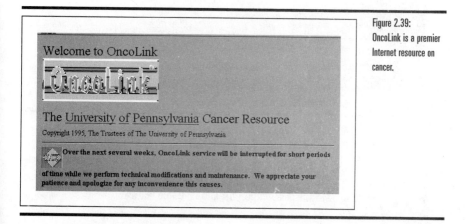

**Figure 2.39:**
OncoLink is a premier Internet resource on cancer.

OncoLink's main menu (see Figure 2.40) has entries for both disease and specialty oriented menus (with entries for just about every form of cancer); for psychological support, cancer organizations, and spirituality; for cancer prevention; for global Internet resources; for a cancer FAQ; and for a billing forum.

The information, written by medical professionals, is primarily targeted toward patients and is presented in clear, easy-to-understand language. "The Nature of Cancer," for example, was written by two oncologists from the University of Pennsylvania Medical School and describes the process of carcinogenesis, the difference between benign and malignant tumors, and the disease process. Other documents cover the role of nutritional support in cancer, chemotherapy, radiation therapy and surgery, and cancer pain management.

Even though many of the Internet's health-related discussion and support groups often cover financial and insurance issues, OncoLink is one of the few informational resources to address the financial aspects and implications of an illness. The OncoLink Billing Forum accepts patient and

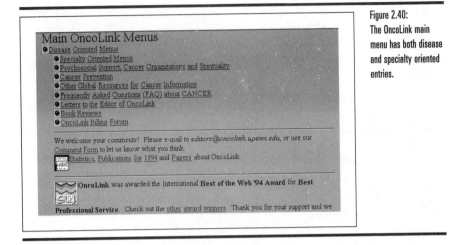

Figure 2.40:
The OncoLink main
menu has both disease
and specialty oriented
entries.

family questions about billing and insurance and returns answers from experts in the health finance field. Because cancer can be financially as well as physically debilitating (and the financial and insurance hassles cause great stress), this is an important and valuable feature.

The links to other Internet resources on cancer are especially comprehensive, with dozens of links to U.S. government resources and to associations, electronic journals and online resources, hospitals, universities, and institutes.

## More...

The Internet has many good cancer resources, more than we can describe in this guide. Here are a few examples.

♦ CANCERGUIDE: A Web site for cancer information devoted to helping you research treatment for your cancer: http://bcn.boulder.co.us/health/cancer/canguide.html.

♦ The Community Breast Health Project, a clearinghouse for breast cancer information and support: http://www-med.stanford.edu/CBHP.

♦ Cancer Medical Discussion Newsgroup: sci.med.diseases.cancer.

OncoLink won a Best of the Web award in 1994, and after a tour of its resources, it's easy to see why!

# Breast Cancer Discussion

BREAST-CANCER

listserv@wvnvm.bitnet

The Breast Cancer discussion list is a very active discussion of all aspects of breast cancer: diagnostic procedures, treatments and procedures, chemotherapy, surgery, radiation treatments, reconstructive surgery, emotional support, and political and social issues. In addition to its well-informed members, some health professionals contribute to the list and add their medical input.

To subscribe, send e-mail to the address above, with the message Subscribe BREAST-CANCER *Yourfirstname Yourlastname*. This is a very busy list, easily averaging 20 to 30 messages a day. BREAST-CANCER now comes in a digest form, but digests currently come every few days rather than daily.

*Don't overdo it when first subscribing to e-mail discussion lists. Some have a very high volume, and you may be deluged with e-mail if you subscribe to even a few of those. Remember to save the list instructions that are sent to you when your subscription is acknowledged, and use the digest command to keep control of busy lists.*

- ◆ Cancer Support Group: alt.support.cancer.

- ◆ Prostate Cancer Support Group: alt.support.cancer.prostate.

- ◆ Support group for people interested in multiple myeloma: http://www.unb.ca/subjects/health/mmee.html.

- ◆ Quick Information about Cancer for Patients and Their Families: http://asa.ugl.lib.umich.edu/chdocs/cancer/CANCERGUIDE.HTML.

## Breast Cancer Information

gopher://nysernet.org/

http://nysernet.org/bcic/default.html

The Breast Cancer Information Clearinghouse (BCIC) is sponsored by the State of New York and NYSERNet and is a comprehensive resource on breast cancer, with plenty of relevant information for people with other types of cancer as well. The BCIC has connections to the Agency for Health Care Policy and Review guidelines on cancer pain management, to the American Cancer Society, to numerous U.S. government resources (including CAN-CERLIT citations and abstracts), and to other related Gopher and Web sites. The BCIC also has numerous documents and fact sheets on breast cancer, including the National Women's Health Report and the *Self* magazine annual breast cancer reports. Here too are archives of the BREAST-CANCER e-mail discussion list and information about the bmt-talk online newsletter on bone marrow transplants.

## CARDIOVASCULAR DISEASE

Cardiovascular disease—heart disease and related problems of the circulatory system—is a major health problem in the U.S. The following Internet areas will help you get in-depth information and discover some supportive resources as well.

## American Heart Association

gopher://gopher.amhrt.org

The American Heart Association (AHA) Gopher is a collection of menus and documents about the AHA, including membership and legislative activities, patient support activities—including support groups and the Heart Healthy information program—information on its research activities, and news bulletins and fact sheets. The AHA Gopher has connections to outside Gopherspace. Watch for future WWW and FTP sites.

*When you find a helpful Web or Gopher resource, be sure to use your hot list or bookmark features to mark the spot so that you can return to it easily.*

# Cardiovascular Information

http://osler.wust/.edu/~murphy/cardiology/compass.html

Cardiology Compass, the Cardiology home page (see Figure 2.41), is a resource for patients and medical professionals that touches on all aspects of cardiology. The page has links to libraries of multimedia images, including heart sounds and murmurs (you'll need special shareware to hear them from your computer), still and video images of ECGs, coronary angiograms, and radiologic images.

Other links include those to the American Heart Association and American College of Cardiology Gophers and to the AHCPR Guidelines mentioned earlier in this book. Look too at the links to Clinical Data and to Clinical Trials, which provides information for stroke patients. Information on acute pericarditis, cardiomyopathy, and hypertension management are provided by links to other Web sites. And, of course, there are links to other cardiology and general Internet health resources.

Especially helpful are the links to the National Heart, Lung, and Blood Institute's (NHLBI) patient education materials, which include smoking and

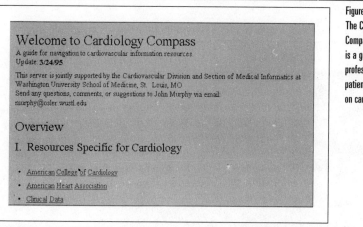

**Figure 2.41:**
The Cardiology Compass Web site is a good source of professional and patient information on cardiology.

Welcome to Cardiology Compass
A guide for navigation to cardiovascular information resources
Update 3/24/95

This server is jointly supported by the Cardiovascular Division and Section of Medical Informatics at Washington University School of Medicine, St. Louis, MO
Send any questions, comments, or suggestions to John Murphy via email:
murphy@osler.wustl.edu

Overview

I. Resources Specific for Cardiology

• American College of Cardiology
• American Heart Association
• Clinical Data

healthy heart questionnaires and fact sheets on coronary heart disease, angina, heart arrhythmia, heart failure, and heart and lung transplants.

## Cardiovascular Diseases

http://128.220.90.135:80/

This Web site at Johns Hopkins Hospital (see Figure 2.42) is primarily for health professionals and for medical education in cardiovascular disease, but if you have a serious heart condition, you likely know enough about your illness and have the medical vocabulary to learn something here. Just be aware that these materials are for a professional, not a patient, audience.

*If you have a serious heart condition, you likely know enough about your illness and have the medical vocabulary to learn something here. Just be aware that these materials are for a professional, not a patient, audience.*

The site, although still "under construction" when we visited, has menu choices for case presentations, tutorials, images and videos, specialists, other resources, and consultations. All the major cardiovascular diseases and treatments are covered.

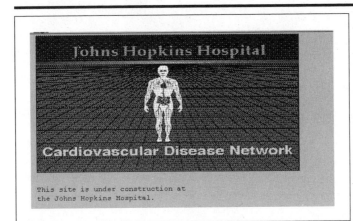

Figure 2.42:
Johns Hopkins Hospital Cardiovascular Disease Network home page has excellent technical information on cardiovascular disease.

# National Heart, Lung, and Blood Institute

gopher://gopher.nhlbi.nih.gov

The National Heart, Lung, and Blood Institute (NHLBI) Gopher is the source for official scientific reports from its task force/working groups on such topics as heart failure, coronary heart disease, and cardiovascular disease prevention.

## More...

If you need information on other diseases and conditions not covered here, check out some of these resources.

- Rare Disease Discussion List, a mailing list for people seeking resources on any rare disorder or wishing to network:
  RARE-DIS
  (listserv@sjuvm.stjohns.edu).

- Multiple Sclerosis Discussion List:
  MSLIST-Ł
  (listerv@technion.bitnet).

- Multiple Sclerosis on the WWW:
  http://www.infosci.org/.

- Amyotrophic Lateral Sclerosis:
  ALS List
  (bro@huey.met.fsu.edu,
  message: personal request).

- Parkinson's Disease Network:
  PARKINSN
  (listserv@vm.utcc.utoronto.ca).

- Stroke Discussion List:
  STROKE-L
  (listserv@ukcc.uky.edu).

- Cystic Fibrosis Discussion and Support:
  CYSTIC FIBROSIS
  (listserv@frmop11.cnusc.fr).

# Looking at Alternative Treatments

Alternative health-care treatments are a popular option for many, whether they're trying to move toward a higher level of wellness or deal with a health concern. A study published in the *New England Journal of Medicine* showed that one-third of the people surveyed had used an "unconventional therapy" within the previous year. That study estimated that Americans may spend as much on alternative health treatments as they do on hospitalizations.

Alternative health treatments are gaining credibility in some medical circles as studies attempt to determine which alternative therapies might work. One attraction is that alternative treatments are often cheaper than conventional medicine. A new institute for the study of alternative medicine has been formed at the National Institutes of Health; its first studies are now underway.

None of this is news to the Internet alternative health community, which has been thriving for some time. Whichever alternative (or "complementary") health treatments pique your interest, you'll likely find a corner of the Internet with people to share information and resources.

This section opens with some general resources and starting points and then explores resources on some individual alternative health systems.

## THE ONLINE ALTERNATIVE HEALTH-CARE REFERENCE SHELF

Check out these comprehensive resources on alternative health care first. These sites and authors have done a lot to organize the Net's alternative health resources for you.

# Dr. Bower's Complementary Medicine

http://galen.med.virginia.edu:80/~pjb3s/ComplementaryHomePage.html

Dr. Bower's home page (see Figure 2.43) is a good place to begin an exploration of alternative health-care Internet resources. Start with the Complementary Practices TOPICS index for articles on and links to the following: acupuncture, Ayurvedic medicine, body/mind medicine, chiropractic, diet and nutrition, energy medicine, flower remedies, herbalist, homeopathy, light therapy, Native American healing, naturopathy, neural tissue testing, neurolinguistic programming, nootropic pharmacology, osteopathy, oxygen therapy, reflexology, reiki, shiatsu, traditional Chinese medicine, and yoga, with more being added all the time.

> *Dr. Bower's home page is a good place to begin an exploration of alternative health-care Internet resources.*

Dr. Bower is also adding a section on current research into complementary therapies (under construction when we visited). The Complementary Medicine page has extensive links to other Internet resources of interest.

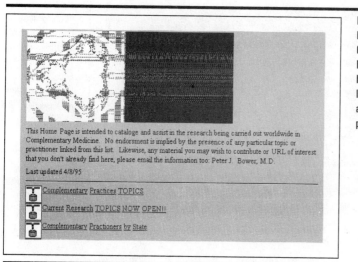

**Figure 2.43:**
Dr. Bower's Complementary Medicine home page has articles on and links to dozens of alternative health-care practices and systems.

## Natural Medicine, Complementary Health Care, and Alternative Therapies

http://www.teleport.com:80/~amrta

This Web site is the home page of the Alchemical Medicine Research and Teaching Association (AMRTA), "a non-profit organization dedicated to the art of healing and the science of medicine." This is a fairly comprehensive collection of resources on alternative health care, with lots to offer practitioners and other health professionals as well as consumers.

Look here for AMRTA's IBIS (Interactive BodyMind Information System) software for alternative practitioners. This is also the home of the PARACEL-SUS mailing list for clinical practitioners interested in alternative health care. AMRTA has links to other Internet health resources and to medical and health organizations and educational institutions.

The Health Information and Tools for Wellness page (see Figure 2.44) has sections on diet and nutrition, understanding ourselves, and medicines and procedures. The overview section has interesting introductory articles on herbs, homeopathy, acupuncture, and holistic health issues and immunity.

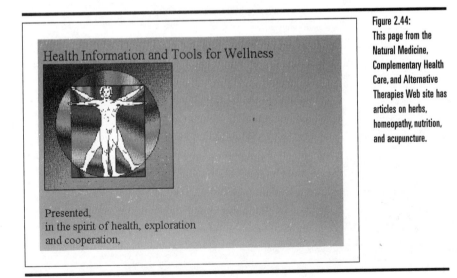

Figure 2.44:
This page from the Natural Medicine, Complementary Health Care, and Alternative Therapies Web site has articles on herbs, homeopathy, nutrition, and acupuncture.

# Alternative Care

http://www.sky.net/~ngt/welcome.html

Alternative Care is a Web newsletter on alternative health care for consumers, practitioners, and students (see Figure 2.45). This page has a definite slant toward chiropractic practice, which should make it especially interesting to some. Resources are eclectic and include online guides to educational programs, student financial aid, improving memory (human not computer), and chiropractic practice marketing. Information sheets and FAQs on a number of alternative therapies (from aromatherapy to Tai Chi) are available too, as is professional information for chiropractors.

This page is linked to the Back page, the Chiropractic page, the Sumeria page, and both Dr. Bower's and the AMRTA pages.

> *Resources are eclectic and include online guides to educational programs, student financial aid, improving memory (human not computer), and chiropractic practice marketing.*

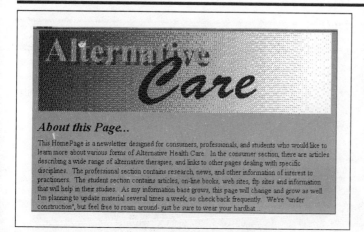

Figure 2.45:
The Alternative Care site is a Web newsletter on alternative health care.

## Alternative Theories and Therapies

http://werple.mira.net.au/sumeria/

Sumeria, a Web site that is part of the Virtual Library, opens its introduction with this statement: "If you think you can detect some bias here, you're probably right." And so it goes from there. Sumeria (see Figure 2.46) is an eclectic collection of information on alternative theories and therapies, from the "conventional" alternatives to those that even the page's author characterizes as "out to lunch." The guiding principle of the site is that all this information needs a home that's accessible; so come for some entertaining and enlightening browsing (just bring a little healthy skepticism to some sections).

*Sumeria is an eclectic collection of information on alternative theories and therapies.*

*If you find your Web browser is taking too long on some of those graphics-heavy home pages, see if it has a feature to delay image retrieval. You can then read the page to see if you're really interested before you spend a lot of time downloading graphics.*

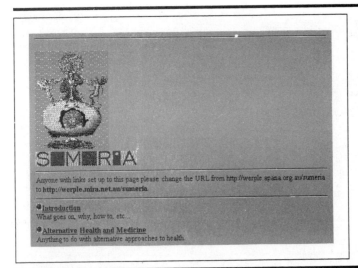

**Figure 2.46:**
Sumeria has an eclectic collection of materials on all kinds of alternative therapies and theories.

# Alternative Health-Care Documents and Questions and Answers

http://sunSITE.sut.ac.jp/arch/academic/medicine/alternative-healthcare

gopher://sunsite.sut.ac.jp/1/academic-info/medicine/alternative-healthcare

The SunSITE archives are the Internet repository for lots of interesting collections, among them an extensive selection of documents and FAQs on alternative health care. Whether you want to read about the health effects of EMFs from power lines, learn about aromatherapy, find out about Essiac (an herbal treatment), or explore ancient Ayurvedic medicine, you can find something of interest—and lots more—here. This archive is a great place to just poke around in for interesting tidbits. There's information on a Kombucha Gopher site, oxygen therapy, the Longevity listserver, and life-enhancement news. Other levels of menus have similar selections and possible hidden treasures.

Our illustration of only one menu (see Figure 2.47) comes from the Web interface. You can also access this resource through Gopher.

**Figure 2.47:**
One of several indexes of documents on alternative health care from the SunSITE Archive.

Index of
/arch/Academic-Info/medicine/alternative-healthcare/

| Name | Last modified | Size | Description |
|------|---------------|------|-------------|
| GUIDE | 23-Apr-95 21:14 | 8K | |
| Herb-Research-Foundat> | 18-Apr-95 06:29 | - | |
| Herb Archives | 22-Apr-95 14:50 | 3K | |
| INDEX | 04-Jan-95 18:55 | 1K | |
| Southwest-School-of-B> | 21-Apr-95 20:47 | - | |
| alternative-medicine/ | 15-Feb-95 20:31 | - | |
| aromatherapy/ | 28-Oct-94 20:09 | - | |
| ayurveda/ | 29-Oct-94 22:01 | - | |
| crystal-healing/ | 05-Apr-95 20:43 | discussion-groups/ 30 | |
| faqs/ 24-Apr-95 20:54 | general/ 19-Apr-95 21:02 | gopher-holes/ | |
| herbs/ 24-Apr-95 20:55 | homeopathy/ 04-Nov-94 23:07 | life-exte | |

## Holistic Health Discusion

HOLISTIC

listserv@siucvmb.bitnet

This is a wide-ranging discussion group, older and more established than wellnesslist (see below). These people discuss all kinds of alternative therapies for all kinds of problems. In just a few days we found questions and responses on Kombucha, the Bates method of eye exercise, yoga, nutrition, supplements, herbs, and more.

To subscribe, send e-mail to the address above, with the message SUB-SCRIBE HOLISTIC *Yourfirstname Yourlastname*. HOLISTIC can be busy sometimes; you may want the digest version.

## Alternative Health Discussion

misc.health.alternative

The misc.health.alternative newsgroup is open to almost any discussion of any and all types of alternative health theories and treatments—from herbalism (and Chinese herbs) to Kombucha, from nutrition to acupuncture to shark

### Business on the Net

Although you might not believe it, the way some on the Internet talk, business is acceptable, and even welcome, on the Internet. The issue for most Net citizens is how and where business is done.

For years the Internet was a commercial-free zone, largely because much of the funding for the network's backbones came from the U.S. government. Most found that policy, called "acceptable use," too restrictive, because it prohibited almost *all* business from using the Net for any purpose. It did, however, sow the seeds for the culture clash on the Internet today.

Most Internet users with any history on the network—and many new users as well—find commercial activity on the Net suspect and find unsolicited advertising abhorrent. As more and more businesses need the Net, however, and as more users like the convenience of having product information (marketing and advertising under another name) and services readily available, some middle ground is emerging. If businesses using the Internet could hold to the following simple cartilage, all the way to urine therapy (yes, urine therapy). There's lots of activity on this newsgroup, which can be fairly contentious at times. The quality of the postings can range from very helpful to dangerous quackery. As with many newsgroups, this one is trying to fend off commercial postings from purveyors of all kinds of alternative products and supplements.

## Wellness Discussion

wellnesslist

majordomo@wellnessmart.com

The wellnesslist discussion is eclectic, covering just about any topic on alternative health nutrition, life extension, fitness, and more. Recommendations of and testimonials for natural health products are common, but the members protest when marketers try to slip in advertising in the guise of a "real" message and in violation of the list's very clear guidelines on commercial activity.

To subscribe, send e-mail to the address above with the message Subscribe wellnesslist. Neither your name nor a subject line is necessary. A digest version of the list is available, which is helpful, because wellnesslist can get fairly busy.

principles, both business and private uses of the Net would probably go more smoothly.

◆ The Net leadership seems to agree that commercial activity—that is, advertising, marketing, retailing, and service provision—can and should be available on the Net.

◆ Businesses should keep advertising off lists and newsgroups if advertising is not part of the expressed purpose of the group.

◆ Advertisers should set up their own Web pages, e-mail, and Gopher servers to deliver their message, product, or service to the people who want to receive it.

◆ Advertisers and businesses should not abuse the privacy of individual mailboxes, mailing lists, or newsgroups.

## Clinical Discussion on Alternative Health Care

PARACELSUS

majordomo@teleport.com

This list is for health-care professionals, in either alternative and/or traditional health care, who want to discuss clinical aspects of alternative health care. Here you'll find practical questions and answers and discourse on theories and modalities of treatment. Interesting discussions, with little "noise." List members must demonstrate some kind of professional involvement in alternative or traditional practice.

*If you find yourself lost in Gopherspace and want to know where you really are, the = sign will detail your position. If you have a Gopher client program, you'll likely have a similar command available to fix your position.*

## ALTERNATIVE HEALTH SYSTEMS

Here's a collection of resources for some of the better-known alternative health systems, theories, and therapies. If you want more in-depth information, many of these resources will point you in the right direction for further research and investigation. If the alternative therapy that you're interested in is not included in this section, use the resources in the Online Alternative Health-Care Reference Shelf above to search for topical information.

## Aromatherapy

http://www.dircon.co.uk:80/home/philrees/fragrant/aroma1.html

Nature's Gifts, Guide to Aromatherapy is clear and accessible, and undoubtedly aromatherapy is one of the most pleasurable of the alternative health systems! This page includes basic descriptions of different methods for using the essential oils (massage, bath, compresses, steam inhalations) and tips for storing and mixing oils. Also included are descriptions of some of the important oils and suggestions for their use (coriander oil for a refreshing and stimulating bath, for example). This appears to be a commercial site, but it does, in the best traditions of the Net, offer a great deal.

# Ayurveda

http://www.protree.com:80/Spirit/ayurveda.html

From the Spirit WWW site comes this paper on Ayurveda (see Figure 2.48). It contains a history of Ayurvedic medicine and its traditions and a discussion of the principles and theories behind it. This is an excellent introduction to this ancient health system from India.

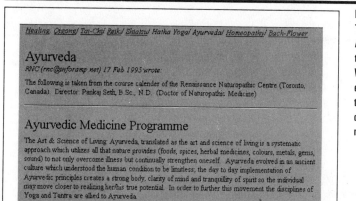

Figure 2.48:
This paper on Ayurvedic medicine, taken from the Spirit WWW site, is an excellent introduction to the history and traditions of an ancient medical system.

# Ayurveda Discussion

alt.health.ayurveda

The Ayurveda newsgroup discusses the principles and practice of Ayurvedic medicine.

# Ayurveda Questions and Answers

ftp://anonymous:@sunsite.unc.edu/pub/academic/medicine/alternative-healthcare/faqs/ayurveda

This site is the home of the alt.health.ayurveda Frequently Asked Questions document.

## Back Pain

ftp://anonymous:@ftp.netcom.com:21/pub/sm/smachado/backpg3.html

Another chiropractic-oriented resource, this site focuses on low back pain (see Figure 2.49) and spine health. It includes information on chiropractic education and institutions and some state regulations. There's lots of interesting activity here (much of it still under construction) and one of the most interesting and extensive sets of links to a wealth of Internet health links all over the world.

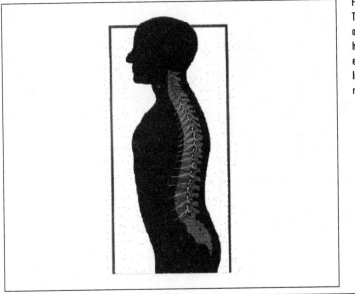

Figure 2.49:
The Back page focuses on back and spine health—and has extensive links to other Internet health resources.

## Chiropractic

http://www.mbnet.mb.ca:80/~jwiens/chiro.html

The Chiropractic page is a central access point for information on chiropractic practice, research, and education. From here you can link to the mailing lists chiro-list and chirosci (chiropractic science and research) and to PARACELSUS and information on educational programs. Research information includes AHCPR research and full text of the AHCPR guidelines on acute lower back pain and other studies and searches of the medical literature on the efficacy of chiropractic treatment. The Chiropractic page also includes links to relevant Internet health resources.

## Chiropractic Discussion

chiro-list

majordomo@silcom.com

This list discusses topics relating to chiropractic theory and practice. To subscribe, send e-mail to the address above with the message subscribe chiro-list. No subject line is necessary.

## Herb Discussion

alt.folklore.herbs

This group discusses a wide-range of topics concerning herbs, herbalism, and herbal uses and treatments. Generally in a query-and-response mode, group members compare notes on effective herbs and doses for various conditions and go over other medicinals (cranberry juice for bladder problems, for example, and the use of tea tree oil in coping with head lice).

## Herbal Discussions

http://www.crl.com/~robbee/herbal.html

Herbal Hall, the Web home of the professional herbalist discussion groups, is a nifty Web and alternative health-care resource. The beautiful botanical graphics put a lot of Web pages to shame, and there's plenty of content and lots of links to boot. Articles and book reviews are presented and updated periodically, including the HERB Article of the Month (see Figure 2.50). Links abound, from the Australian National Botanic Garden to the Medicinal Herb Garden to the FDA and the Medical Herbalist newsletter. The page also has a link to the Herbal Hall FTP resource files and an image bank of herb images.

> *The beautiful botanical graphics put a lot of Web pages to shame.*

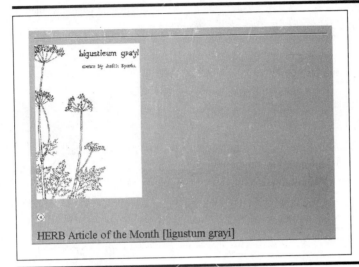

HERB Article of the Month [ligustum grayi]

**Figure 2.50:**
This image of *ligustum grayi* is from the HERB Article of the Month in the Herbal Hall Web page.

## Herb Research

http://sunsite.unc.edu:80/hrf/

This Web site from the Herbal Research Foundation takes the form of an online publication with feature "articles" and a collection of photographic images of herbs. If you're traveling, you can check out an article on herbs to pack in your bag or read an article on two herbs thought to boost immune function (see Figure 2.51)

## Homeopathic Resources

ftp://antenna.apc.org/homeo/resource.lst

This site contains a collection of Internet resources on homeopathy, including many libraries, databases, software, and archives not included in other Net homeopathic pointers. It is updated regularly.

Figure 2.51:
Read an article on
herbs and immunity
from the Herb Research
News Web page.

## Boosting Immunity With Herbs

**by Rob McCaleb, HRF President**

For over 4,000 years, the Chinese have used certain herbs to prevent common diseases. The ancient Chinese knew nothing of bacteria or viruses, yet some of these herbs were said to "strengthen the exterior", or the "shield". Modern scientific research is confirming that they were right. Thousands of years later, and sixty years after the discovery of penicillin, the study of herbs affecting the immune system is one of the hottest topics in pharmacological research. Can herbs really strengthen our resistance and help us lead healthier lives? Both the wisdom of centuries of observation, and the scrutiny of the scientific laboratory, support the view that they can.

### HOW THE IMMUNE SYSTEM WORKS

Our immune system recognizes and destroys anything foreign to the body, including cells like bacteria and other microbes, and foreign particles including toxic compounds. This recognition and destruction is performed by cells in the circulatory and the lymphatic systems. These cells are produced in the

# Homeopathy Discussion

HOMEOPATHY

homeopathy-request@dungeon.com

The Homeopathy discussion list is home to serious students of homeopathy, but they are amazingly polite and helpful to newcomers with questions. If you're not at home with the fairly technical vocabulary of homeopathy, this list may read like a foreign language, but some respectful lurking and research into other Internet resources may help clue you in. List members are uncomfortable giving personal or specific medical advice; this is a place to learn about a system, not seek a diagnosis.

Homeopathy has a fairly heavy volume. To subscribe, send e-mail to homeopathy-request@dungeon.com with the message subscribe. No subject is necessary. To get the digest, send the subscribe message to homeopathy-d-request@dungeon.com. Again, no subject.

# Homeopathy Information

http://www.dungeon.com:80/home/cam/homeo.html

The Homeopathy home page (see Figure 2.52) is the jumping-off point for Internet resources on homeopathy. Start here for links to the Homeopathy FAQ, the Homeopathy and HOLISTIC e-mail discussion lists, and addresses of homeopathic resources in the U.S., in the UK, and worldwide. Resources for practitioners include software, the HomeoNet service, and a link to PARACELSUS. The page also links to some commercial resources that might be useful and, of course, to a range of Internet health resources, including Complementary Medicine, AMRTA, the Yahoo Health : Alternative Medicine directory, and the Midwifery, Pregnancy and Birth-Related Information Index.

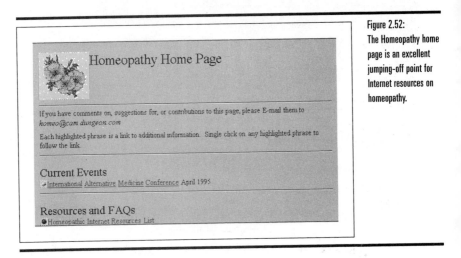

**Figure 2.52:**
The Homeopathy home page is an excellent jumping-off point for Internet resources on homeopathy.

## Homeopathy Questions and Answers

ftp://sunsite.unc.edu/pub/academic/medicine/alternative-healthcare/faqs/homeopathy

This is the home of the Homeopathy FAQ for those without Web access. The Homeopathy FAQ is also available on the Homeopathy Web page at http://www.dungeon.com:80/home/cam/homeo.html (see Figure 2.53).

## Medicinal and Aromatic Plants Discussion

herb@trearn.bitnet

The Herb list covers herbal medicine and related topics. Generally, the posts are requests for help and responses to questions on herbal medicine, preparations for use and dosages, sources and uses of herbs, side effects of herbal

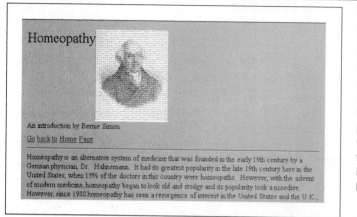

Homeopathy

An introduction by Bernie Simon

Go back to Home Page

Homeopathy is an alternative system of medicine that was founded in the early 19th century by a German physician, Dr. Hahnemann. It had its greatest popularity in the late 19th century here in the United States, when 15% of the doctors in this country were homeopaths. However, with the advent of modern medicine, homeopathy began to look old and stodgy and its popularity took a nosedive. However, since 1980 homeopathy has seen a resurgence of interest in the United States and the U.K.,

Figure 2.53:
A version of the Homeopathy FAQ illustrated with the visage of Samuel Hahnemann, the father of homeopathy, can be found on the Homeopathy Web page. The plain vanilla version is posted on the homeopathy mailing list and available by FTP.

preparations, and more. Messages are usually short and to the point (a refreshing change from some lists and groups), with little evidence of flaming, proselytizing, or unwanted commercial activity (another refreshing change).

To subscribe, send e-mail to the address above, with the message subscribe *Yourfirstname Yourlastname.* No subject line is necessary.

# Naturopathy

http://www.sims.net/organizations/naturopath/naturopath.html

The Naturopathy home page is a central spot for access to the naturopathy mailing list and to the naturopathy newsletter and its archive files.

*Resources on the Net can move around a lot. If you find that a URL or location listed in this book no longer works for a resource you're interested in, check some of the main Web or Gopher sites first for clues to its whereabouts. Relevant FAQs, newsgroups, and mailing lists are also good places to look for new addresses or URLs. If all else fails (and only when all else has failed), post a query to the one newsgroup or list that most closely matches the topic of the missing resource.*

## Oriental Medicine Discussion

OrMed

listserv@bkhouse.cts.com

The OrMed mailing list is "dedicated to the discussion of Oriental Medicine in all its forms, including acupuncture, herbs, massage, breathwork, exercise and more." The list owner aims at a friendly and positive discussion and says the membership includes nationally known practitioners, writers in the field, a few acupuncture students, and many people just interested in oriental medicine. Individual requests for help with health problems are discouraged (over-the-Net diagnosis doesn't work in any health-care modality).

To subscribe to OrMed mailing list, send e-mail to listserv@bkhouse.cts.com with the message SUBSCRIBE Your e-mail@address OrMed. No subject line is required; any will be fine. To get a help file and instructions for getting the OrMed FAQ, send the command HELP to the listserv address.

## Oriental Medicine Resources

ftp://anonymous:@ftp.cts.com:21/pub/nkraft/ormed.html

The Oriental Medicine home page is the Web home of the OrMed mailing list, with easy access to the FAQ, the list archives, and an archive of articles by list members. The page also links you to some standard and not-so-standard Internet health resources, including the Homeopathy and Herbal Hall Web pages, the National Library of Medicine, and the Visible Human Project.

## Osteopathy

http://www.demon.co.uk:80/osteopath/index.html

Osteopathic medicine is more mainstream than "alternative," but this Web site is a good introduction to the principles of osteopathy and some important resources. You can review the osteopathic philosophy, check out *The Osteopath*, a quarterly print and electronic journal, and review the status of osteopathy around the world. There are links to information about schools, practitioners, products, and services and to the usual interesting mixed bag of other Internet health resources.

# Qigong

/http://www.protree.com:80/Spirit/qigong.html

Qigong is the meditative practice and belief system behind the more familiar Tai Chi Chuan and King Fu. This page (see Figure 2.54) from the Spirit WWW site gives a clear and interesting description of Qigong and its positive health effects and goes into the work of Qigong master Yan Xin, including some fairly startling claims. References and bibliography of both English and Chinese sources are included.

Healing Qigong/ Tai-Chi/ Reiki/ Shiatsu/ Hatha Yoga/ Ayurveda/ Homeopathy/ Bach-Flower

## Yan Xin Qigong
A Brief Introduction To Yan Xin Qigong
International Yan Xin Qigong Association

Frank Zhu (fan@dggp12.chem.purdue.edu) 28 Jun 1994 writes:

## WHAT IS QIGONG?

To begin with, the word "Qigong" (pronounced as Chee-Gong) is created by combining two characters in Chinese. The first character, "Qi," literally air, represents a flowing material of energy that exists in everything and permeates the universe. Related concept in English that approximate the rich connotations of the Chinese character Qi is "bio-energy." Through a method or practice, people can learn to interact and utilize the universal energy that exists around, and within, them. This methodology is called "Gong." The Chinese character "gong" represents the effort placed into Qi practice as well as the power gained through such practice. In other words, Qigong literally means "the meditation practice of Qi energy". In America, during the last twenty-five years, people have become familiar with Chinese practices that are related to Qigong.

Figure 2.54:
A paper on Qigong and the work of Yan Xin, taken from the Spirit WWW site

# Tai Chi Chuan

http://www.protree.com:80/Spirit/tai-chi.html

Another paper from the Spirit WWW site, this one discusses Tai Chi Chuan as a system of health enhancement and exercise, as well as a martial art.

# Staying Emotionally Healthy

Although some in science may dispute the body-mind connection (though fewer every year), most of us realize all too clearly that we can't be truly fit and feel well if our emotional health is in disarray or our mental state is crumbling. The Internet has a wide range of resources on emotional health, mental health, psychology, and psychiatry. Some are immediately helpful in our everyday lives; other resources are targeted to researchers and scholars in the field but still may have some usefulness for lay people.

In addition to the information resources, the Internet sometimes seems like a vast support group; and certainly there *are* plenty of online support groups to join. Whatever your problem or issue, it's likely you can find an existing support group—either a newsgroup or an e-mail discussion list—of people who share your problems and will lend you a helping hand.

This section starts with general resources and Internet-wide resource indexes and concludes with resources for specific mental health concerns.

## THE ONLINE MENTAL-HEALTH REFERENCE SHELF

As with so much of the Internet, hard-working, helpful, and well-informed folks (most of them volunteers) have gone before you, locating interesting and rewarding resources and organizing them into usable indexes. Start with these general resources and indexes to the Internet's resources on mental health and psychology.

## Psychology Around the World

http://rs1.cc.und.nodak.edu:80/misc/jBAT/psychres.html

This is a wonderful collection of links to resources on all aspects of emotional health, psychology, and psychiatry, mostly in the U.S. but some international ones as well (see Figure 2.55). Topic-focused links include the Alzheimer's Web, Facts for Families, Drug-Related Information, Eating Disorders, Mood Disorders, Emotional Support on the Internet, and Sexual Assault Information. There are links to organizations—American Psychology Association and the American Psychiatry Association—and to institutions, including Purdue, the University of North Dakota, Yale, and the University of Wisconsin-Milwaukee. Links to publications include Psycoloquy, Psychiatry Online, Psyche, and several journals on behavior analysis.

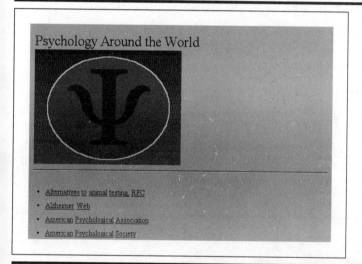

Psychology Around the World

- Alternatives to animal testing, RFC
- Alzheimer Web
- American Psychological Association
- American Psychological Society

Figure 2.55:
Psychology Around the World organizes a wealth of Internet mental health and psychology resources into a comprehensive set of Web links.

# Psychology Resources on the Web

http://www.tezcat.com:80/~tina/psych.pages/grohol.web-pointers.html

Here is another good starting point for finding mental health resources on the Internet. John M. Grohol has organized some excellent links to Web resources. You can jump from here to links such as the Al-Anon/Alateen Web page, Psychiatry Online, Patient Advocacy Phone Numbers, InterPsych, HabitSmart, and the Attention Deficit Disorder page.

## Mental Health

http://www.cc.emory.edu:80/WHSCL/medweb.mentalhealth.html

MedWeb is yet another comprehensive index to Web mental health and psychology resources. MedWeb has more substance-abuse related links than the others, including Cocaine Anonymous and the Join Together Gopher and links to services at the National Clearinghouse for Alcohol and Drug Information.

## American Psychological Association

http://www.apa.org

gopher://gopher.apa.org

PsychNET™ (see Figure 2.56) is the American Psychological Association's (APA) Internet presence. Although the material is primarily of interest to psychology professionals and APA members, material of interest to the rest of us appears here, including journal tables of contents (if you're doing research), articles from periodicals, reviews, and more.

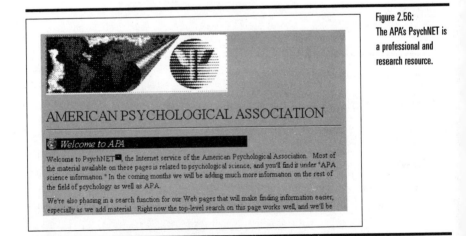

Figure 2.56:
The APA's PsychNET is a professional and research resource.

# Psycoloquy

http://www.w3.org:80/hypertext/DataSources/bySubject/Psychology/Psycoloquy.html

PSYC
listserv@pucc.princeton.edu

sci.psychology.digest

Psycoloquy is an online professional journal sponsored by the American Psychology Association. It is refereed, which means that the articles undergo scholarly review by the association's editorial board before they are posted.

## EMOTIONAL WELLNESS

Staying well emotionally often means coping with personal issues before they escalate into big problems. Here's a selection of Internet resources that might be helpful.

## Self-Help Psychology Magazine

http://www.well.com/ user/self-help

This is an online popular psychology magazine, just like those on the newsstand. *Self-Help* (see Figure 2.57) has feature articles ("Should You Be Concerned about Your Drinking?"), book and product reviews, and departments with helpful articles ("Avoiding Workaholism" and "Spicing Up Your Sex Life," for example) on such topics as relationships, sexuality, addictions and tobacco, parenting and family life, men's issues, depression and anxiety, health, lesbian/gay/bisexual issues, and work and finances. All the

*All the departments and articles shown on the home page are free and accessible.*

departments and articles shown on the home page are free and accessible; other features, such as classifieds, are for paying subscribers only. There's a growing set of Internet psychology links as well.

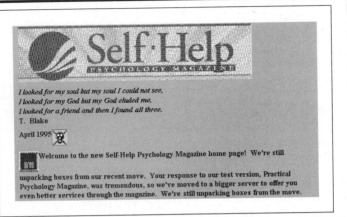

Figure 2.57:
*Self Help Psychology Magazine* brings a readable popular psychology magazine to you online.

## Mental Health Maintenance

*gopher://oasis.cc.purdue.edu*

For some good, clearly written fact sheets on maintaining positive emotional health and coping with common problems, check out the Mental Health menu at the student health services Gopher at Purdue. Written for a college-age audience, the information—on eating disorders, alcohol awareness, quitting smoking, and more—is useful for all ages.

## Facts for Families

*http://www.med.umich.edu:80/aacap/facts.index.html*

Facts for Families (see Figure 2.58) is an online service of the American Academy of Child and Adolescent Psychiatry (AACAP), which contains the complete text of the academy's series of information sheets on emotional and psychological issues facing children and families. Topics range from common issues, such as discipline, step-family problems, and learning disabilities, to more serious concerns. Ordering information for printed copies is included.

> *Topics range from common issues, such as discipline, step-family problems, and learning disabilities, to more serious concerns.*

Figure 2.58:
Facts for Families has information on emotional and psychological issues facing children and families.

## PUBLIC INFORMATION

"Facts for Families" to educate parents and families about psychiatric disorders affecting children and adolescents, the Academy publishes these 46 information sheets which provide concise and up-to-date material on issues such as the depressed child, teen suicide, stepfamily problems and child sexual abuse. Cited and recommended by such publications as Better Homes & Gardens and USA Today. (Fact sheets #1-29 are available in Spanish.) $15.00 for the complete set of 46, single sheet free with self-addressed, stamped envelope. Bulk orders $.25 per sheet. Order: PIFFF-___ (FILL IN APPROPRIATE NUMBERS LISTED BELOW). Please mail your order to: AACAP
Attn: PUBLIC INFORMATION
3615 Wisconsin Avenue, NW
Washington, DC 20016

#1- Children and Divorce
#2- Teenagers with Eating Disorders
#3- Teens; Alcohol and Other Drugs
#4- The Depressed Child
#5- Child Abuse: The Hidden Bruises
#6- Children Who Can't Pay Attention

# Children, Youth, and Family

gopher://tinman.mes.umn.edu.

The Children Youth and Family Consortium Electronic Clearinghouse is an excellent resource on family-life issues—everything about children and family relationships. You'll find information and articles on adoption, infertility, children with special needs, kids and media (see Figure 2.59), and parenting and child-care issues. There's also a section called FatherNet, with the Father's Resource Center and articles of interest.

Figure 2.59:
The Children Youth and Family Consortium Electronic Clearinghouse has helpful articles for parents, such as this one titled "TV Violence: What Parents Can Do."

```
Acting Against Violence
TV Violence: What Parents Can Do
10 Tips from the Experts

The Academy, The American Psychological Association (APA) and the
Center for Media Education give the following recommendations on
how parents can best control family television viewing.

Children Youth and Family Consortium Electronic Clearinghouse.
Permission is granted to create and distribute copies of this
document for noncommercial purposes provided that the author and
CYFCEC receive acknowledgment and this notice is included.  Phone
(612) 626-1212 EMAIL: cyfcec@maroon.tc.umn.edu

Only on TV is there violence without pain. Sometimes TV violence
is even supposed to be funny.  But grown-ups know that real
violence causes lots of pain and sadness.

Just as children learn from their older brothers and sisters, they
also learn from their television heroes.  Some children who watch
lots of violence on TV learn to fight more.  Others learn to
become victims.  And many learn that violence is fun to watch,
even in real life.  These kids encourage their friends to fight.
```

## Grief, Death, and Dying

gopher://gopher.rivendell.org

GriefNet is an online resource on grief, bereavement, death, and dying. The Gopher has regional and national resource listings, information on hospices, educational programs, media resources, topical articles, and more. One article in a menu on natural and human disasters, for example, is titled "What to Tell Children about Terrorist Bombings." GriefNet also sponsors a series of e-mail discussions: grief-chat (see below), grief-parents, grief-training, and grief-widows.

## Emotional Support

http://asa.ugl.lib.umich.edu:80/chdocs/support/emotion.html

The Emotional Support Guide (see Figure 2.60) Web page is an excellent pointer to Internet resources concerning grief and bereavement and support for physical loss and chronic illness. The page has links to resources and indexes to resources by both title and the Internet tool used.

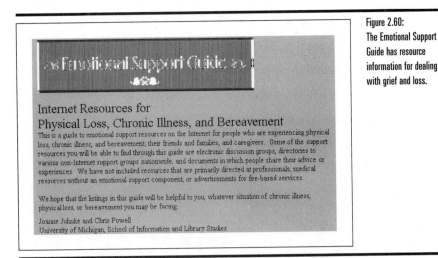

**Figure 2.60:**
The Emotional Support Guide has resource information for dealing with grief and loss.

# Grief Discussion

grief-chat

majordomo@falcon.ic.net

The grief-chat list (from GriefNet) is for "general discussion on anything related to grief, bereavement, death, dying, or any other major loss." To subscribe, send e-mail to the above address with the message subscribe grief-chat *Yourname@e-mail address*. No subject line is necessary.

## SUBSTANCE ABUSE

Problems with alcohol, drugs, and tobacco can be an enormous burden to individuals and to their families and friends. Here are a few places on the Internet to get help and information.

# AA Information

http://www.moscow.com:80/Resources/SelfHelp/AA/

A Web site for Alcoholics Anonymous information (though not sponsored by AA), this page has reams of public domain AA documents and articles and AA organizational information. The original 1939 version of the book *Alcoholics Anonymous* is available, as are pamphlets and brochures, shareware, and photos of AA founders Bill W. and Dr. Bob. This site includes links to other recovery sites on the Internet.

# Al-Anon and Alateen

http://solar.rtd.utk.edu/~al-anon/

This Web site (see Figure 2.61) is for families and friends of alcoholics. The Al-Anon and Alateen page includes the Twelve Steps and Twelve Traditions, plus a 20-item questionnaire to see if Al-Anon is right for you. Information on finding an Al-Anon or Alateen group is also included.

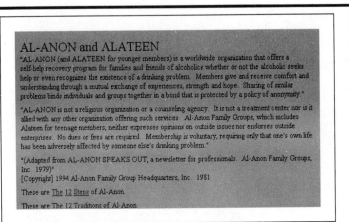

AL-ANON and ALATEEN

"AL-ANON (and ALATEEN for younger members) is a worldwide organization that offers a self-help recovery program for families and friends of alcoholics whether or not the alcoholic seeks help or even recognizes the existence of a drinking problem. Members give and receive comfort and understanding through a mutual exchange of experiences, strength and hope. Sharing of similar problems binds individuals and groups together in a bond that is protected by a policy of anonymity."

"AL-ANON is not a religious organization or a counseling agency. It is not a treatment center nor is it allied with any other organization offering such services. Al-Anon Family Groups, which includes Alateen for teenage members, neither expresses opinions on outside issues nor endorses outside enterprises. No dues or fees are required. Membership is voluntary, requiring only that one's own life has been adversely affected by someone else's drinking problem."

"(Adapted from AL-ANON SPEAKS OUT, a newsletter for professionals. Al-Anon Family Groups, Inc. 1979)"
[Copyright] 1994 Al-Anon Family Group Headquarters, Inc. 1981

These are The 12 Steps of Al-Anon.

These are The 12 Traditions of Al-Anon.

**Figure 2.61:**
The Al-Anon and Alateen Web site has resources for family members and friends of alcoholics.

## AA Recovery Support

alt.recovery.aa

This online support group is in the AA mode for those in recovery. Generally, you'll find very helpful and supportive posts on a variety of topics of interest to those recovering from alcoholism.

## National Clearinghouse for Alcohol and Drug Information

http://www.health.org:80/

telnet:// ncadi.health.org

The National Clearinghouse for Alcohol and Drug Information (NCADI) Web page (see Figure 2.62) is a good central spot for information on substance abuse and substance abuse prevention, with information and resources on alcohol, drugs, and tobacco. You can get copies of U.S. government reports, including the *National Household Survey on Drug Abuse* and the *Prevention Primer*. Links to other substance-abuse-related Internet resources include Join Together, the Partnerships Against Violence Network (PAVNET), and the Higher Education Center for Alcohol and Other Drug Prevention. You can also use Telnet to access NCADI's PREVLINE Bulletin Board.

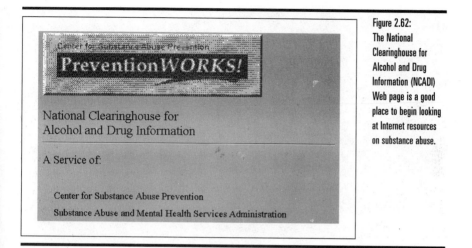

Figure 2.62:
The National
Clearinghouse for
Alcohol and Drug
Information (NCADI)
Web page is a good
place to begin looking
at Internet resources
on substance abuse.

## Drug Information Resources

http://www.pitt.edu:80/~mbtst3/druginfo.html

This site contains links to and resources on drugs and drug politics. It's definitely more from the drug *culture* than from the drug *treatment* point of view. It has pointers to newsgroups and links to Web, Telnet, and FTP resources.

## MENTAL HEALTH

Emotional problems and mental illness are serious concerns that warrant real help, usually professional help at that. After you've set that process in motion, here are some resources and support groups to help you.

## Anxiety/Panic Support Group

alt.support.anxiety-panic

This online support group is for sufferers of anxiety and panic attacks. Discussions focus on causes, treatments, and related physical conditions. Medications are also a big topic, as is general support.

## About Flame Wars

The terms *flame wars* and *flaming* refer to a form of verbal aggression that takes place in the online world, beginning when one party or another takes grievous offense at a newsgroup posting or an e-mail list message. Unfortunately, a one-way flame is a rare occurrence. Usually flame wars escalate into all-out verbal conflict between at least the two initial parties; often more and more readers can't help but join the melee by throwing in their two cents' worth (or more ) of flames.

And, all the while, the rest of the newsgroup or mailing list are innocent but irritated bystanders, having to read or, at least, delete the rants and raves of the flamers. Flame wars can be relatively tame exchanges of nasty verbal barbs or all out nuclear war with the vilest profanity. Either way, it isn't pleasant to read (especially if you pay for Internet access, pay long-distance charges, or have e-mail expenses), and it is a real waste of network resources.

How to avoid it? First, don't ask for trouble. Many consider an unsolicited commercial posting to be just cause for a mega-flame. Spamming—posting the same (usually commercial, meaningless, or just inane) message across numerous

## Attention Deficit Disorder

http://www.seas.upenn.edu:80/~mengwong/add/

ftp://ftp.netcom.com:/pub/ld/lds/add/

This archive is a comprehensive collection of Net resources on attention deficit disorder (ADD). Here you'll find lots of articles (both technical and nontechnical), official diagnostic criteria and simple screening tests (with appropriate warnings about self-diagnosis), and tips for coping with ADD as an adult (see Figure 2.63), as a family member, or as the parent of an ADD child. The ADD FAQ is here. You'll also find information on medications and pointers to online support groups.

groups—is also flame bait. And some consider it their mission to educate erring newbies by singeing their eyebrows.

Second, watch your Net manners. Be careful of sarcasm or witticisms gone wrong. Don't use all caps in your messages. Don't send an unsubscribe message to an entire mailing list of 1000 people.

Third, turn the other cheek. If you are being flamed, just ignore it. If you feel you just can't let it go by, respond to the person, not to the whole list or newsgroup. If you're tempted to join another's fray, resist. You won't make things any better, and you'll probably make them worse. If the flaming doesn't subside, and you can't tolerate another nasty exchange, send a message to the list owner asking him or her to cool things down. Or just unsubscribe until it all passes.

Finally, respect the topics and philosophies of the groups as they exist. Don't send messages extolling the virtues of meat-eating to a vegetarian mailing list, for example, or don't otherwise offend group sensibilities. If you find you don't agree with the content or tone of a given group, just don't join in.

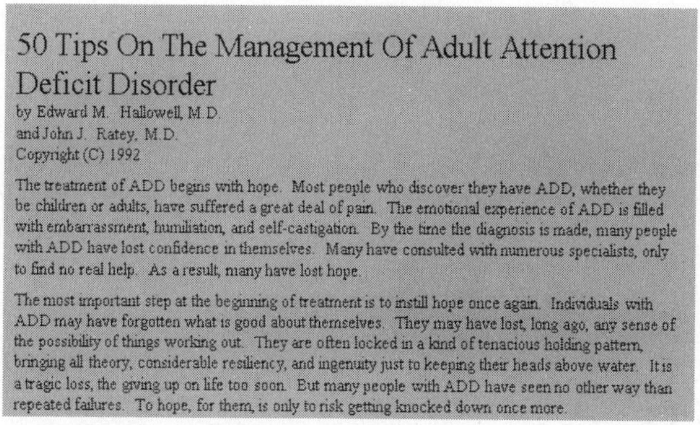

## 50 Tips On The Management Of Adult Attention Deficit Disorder

by Edward M. Hallowell, M.D.
and John J. Ratey, M.D.
Copyright (C) 1992

The treatment of ADD begins with hope. Most people who discover they have ADD, whether they be children or adults, have suffered a great deal of pain. The emotional experience of ADD is filled with embarrassment, humiliation, and self-castigation. By the time the diagnosis is made, many people with ADD have lost confidence in themselves. Many have consulted with numerous specialists, only to find no real help. As a result, many have lost hope.

The most important step at the beginning of treatment is to instill hope once again. Individuals with ADD may have forgotten what is good about themselves. They may have lost, long ago, any sense of the possibility of things working out. They are often locked in a kind of tenacious holding pattern, bringing all theory, considerable resiliency, and ingenuity just to keeping their heads above water. It is a tragic loss, the giving up on life too soon. But many people with ADD have seen no other way than repeated failures. To hope, for them, is only to risk getting knocked down once more.

Figure 2.63:
This article from the Attention Deficit Disorder Archives offers coping tips for adults with attention deficit disorder.

# Adults with Attention Deficit Disorder Discussion

ADDULT

LISTSERV@SJUVM.BITNET

ADDULT is a very active discussion list for adults with Attention Deficit Disorder. Topics include coping strategies, dealing with work and family, diagnosis, medications, and treatment.

To subscribe, send e-mail to the address above with the message SUBSCRIBE ADDULT *Yourfirstname Yourlastname*. No subject line is required.

# Parents of Children with ADD Discussion

add-parents

majordomo@mv.mv.com

This attention deficit disorder discussion is for parents of children with the disorder. To subscribe, send e-mail to the address above, with the message subscribe add-parents. No subject or name is required.

# Depression Resources

http://www.duke.edu:80/~ntd/depression.html

This Web site on depression has pointers to relevant newsgroups and to the Walkers-in-Darkness e-mail discussion list. You can find the Depression FAQ here as well.

*If you're concerned about joining an Internet emotional support newsgroup or discussion list because you must keep your situation absolutely private, investigate one of the anonymous mail forwarders. For information on the best-known mail forwarder (in Finland), send mail to help@anon.penet.fi.*

# Eating Disorders

http://ccwf.cc.utexas.edu:80/jackson/UTHealth/eating.html

This document (see Figure 2.64), from the University of Texas, is an excellent and clearly written basic discussion of eating disorders. The author

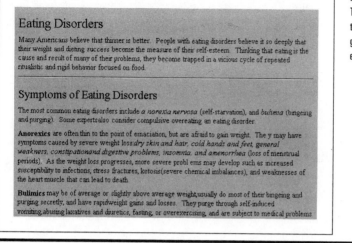

Figure 2.64:
This fact sheet from the University of Texas gives the basics on eating disorders.

## Eating Disorders

Many Americans believe that thinner is better. People with eating disorders believe it so deeply that their weight and dieting success become the measure of their self-esteem. Thinking that eating is the cause and result of many of their problems, they become trapped in a vicious cycle of repeated ritualistic and rigid behavior focused on food.

### Symptoms of Eating Disorders

The most common eating disorders include *anorexia nervosa* (self-starvation), and *bulimia* (bingeing and purging). Some experts also consider compulsive overeating an eating disorder.

**Anorexics** are often thin to the point of emaciation, but are afraid to gain weight. They may have symptoms caused by severe weight loss: *dry skin and hair, cold hands and feet, general weakness, constipation and digestive problems, insomnia, and amenorrhea* (loss of menstrual periods). As the weight loss progresses, more severe problems may develop such as increased susceptibility to infections, stress fractures, ketosis (severe chemical imbalances), and weaknesses of the heart muscle that can lead to death.

**Bulimics** may be of average or slightly above average weight, usually do most of their bingeing and purging secretly, and have rapid weight gains and losses. They purge through self-induced vomiting, abusing laxatives and diuretics, fasting, or overexercising, and are subject to medical problems

discusses the types of eating disorders and the symptoms, with questions to evaluate the seriousness of the problem. Strategies for controlling eating disorders are offered, including some special notes for athletes.

## Mental Illness Discussion

MADNESS

listserv@sjuvm.stjohns.edu

The MADNESS list is an e-mail discussion list for "people who experience mood swings, fright, voices, and visions." It's intended to be a forum for sharing information and discussing ways to change the social systems that impact its members. To subscribe, send e-mail to the address above with the message SUBSCRIBE MADNESS *Yourfirstname Yourlastname*. No subject line is needed.

## Mood Disorders

http://avocado.pc.helsinki.fi:80/~janne/mood/mood.html

This helpful Web site has resources on and links to areas that primarily focus on depression. You can get the Depression FAQ, review a couple of self-assessment scales for mania and depression, review literature on common prescription drugs for depression (supplied by the pharmaceutical companies), and read articles on serotonin, tricyclic antidepressants, and important food-drug interactions. You'll find links to the <u>Winter Depression (Seasonal Affective Disorder)</u> page and other resources on SAD, to the <u>OCD</u> (Obsessive Compulsive Disorder) server, and to <u>Pendulum Resources</u> (which deals with bipolar disorder).

## Cyclical Affective Disorders

pendulum

majordomo@ucar.edu

The Pendulum mailing list is a support group for people with bipolar depression or another cyclical affective disorder. Discussions range over issues of drugs and drug treatments, side effects, going on and off medications, relationships with family and friends, job, the mental health profession, and dealing with the drastic swings toward manic or suicidal behavior.

Pendulum is an incredibly busy list. Be sure to get the digest version unless you have a lot of time to deal with your e-mail.

To subscribe, send an e-mail message to the address above with the message subscribe pendulum. No subject line is necessary.

## Depression Discussion

walkers

walkers@world.std.com.

The Walkers-in-Darkness (aka Bearers-of-Light) is an e-mail discussion list on all forms of depression. The list is intended for families and friends as well as for depression sufferers themselves. Walkers provide support for one another and share coping strategies and information on medications and treatments. The tone is generally very supportive, often with a real sense that people are watching out for one another. This is a *very busy* list (with two daily digests), obviously filling a big need for its members.

*Walkers provide support for one another and share coping strategies and information on medications and treatments.*

To subscribe, send e-mail to the address above with the message subscribe walkers. No name or subject line is required. Review the response letter you get from the list owner to get the list overview and instructions for the digest version and anonymous posting.

# Seasonal Affective Disorder

http://avocado.pc.helsinki.fi:80/~janne/mood/sad.html

Visit this Winter Depression (see Figure 2.65) Web page for coping tips and sound counsel (some of it historical) on dealing with light-deprivation-induced winter depression. You'll find pointers to helpful products, organizations, and reading.

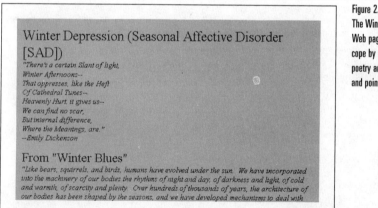

**Figure 2.65:**
The Winter Depression Web page helps you cope by providing poetry and helpful tips and pointers.

Winter Depression (Seasonal Affective Disorder [SAD])

"There's a certain Slant of light,
Winter Afternoons--
That oppresses, like the Heft
Of Cathedral Tunes--
Heavenly Hurt, it gives us--
We can find no scar,
But internal difference,
Where the Meanings, are."
--Emily Dickenson

From "Winter Blues"

"Like bears, squirrels, and birds, humans have evolved under the sun. We have incorporated into the machinery of our bodies the rhythms of night and day, of darkness and light, of cold and warmth, of scarcity and plenty. Over hundreds of thousands of years, the architecture of our bodies has been shaped by the seasons, and we have developed mechanisms to deal with

*Avoid chiming in with "me too" messages that just crowd everyone's in-boxes without adding to the discussion. Try not to post to a group or a list unless you have something substantive to add to the conversation.*

# ONLINE SUPPORT

No matter what you're going through, you can probably find a support group of people who understand somewhere out on the Internet. In addition to the resources detailed in this section, many, many more newsgroups and e-mail discussion lists are out there. Try some of these resources first. If you still can't find the right group for you, perhaps you can start one of your own!

# Psychology Support Groups

http://chat.carleton.ca/~tscholbe/psych.html

This helpful list of pointers to online support groups (see Figure 2.66) is maintained by John M. Grohol and posted regularly to a number of newsgroups and mailing lists. You can also pick up a copy at the Web URL above.

## More . . .

Here are just some of the many support groups. If you don't see what you need, get John M. Grohol's support newsgroup pointer described above.

- ◆ Recovering from abuse:
  alt.abuse.recovery

- ◆ Dealing with abuse:
  alt.abuse.transcendence

- ◆ General recovery:
  alt.recovery

- ◆ Recovering from sexual abuse:
  alt.sexual.abuse.recovery

- ◆ Attention deficit disorders:
  alt.support.attn-deficit

- ◆ Learning disabilities:
  alt.support.learning-disab

- ◆ Loneliness:
  alt.support.loneliness

- ◆ Schizophrenia:
  alt.support.schizophrenia

- ◆ Shyness:
  alt.support.shyness

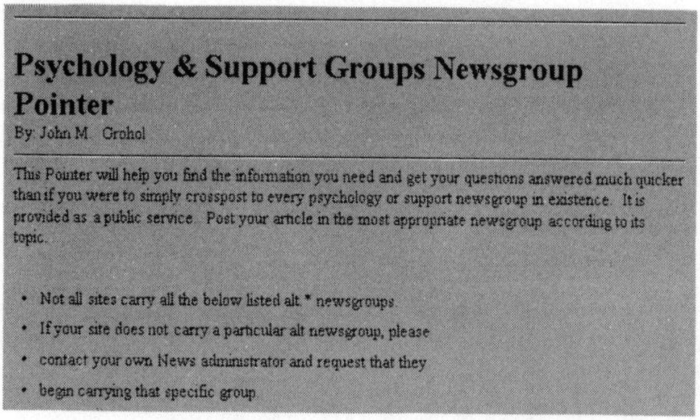

## Psychology & Support Groups Newsgroup Pointer

By: John M. Grohol

This Pointer will help you find the information you need and get your questions answered much quicker than if you were to simply crosspost to every psychology or support newsgroup in existence. It is provided as a public service. Post your article in the most appropriate newsgroup according to its topic.

- Not all sites carry all the below listed alt.* newsgroups.
- If your site does not carry a particular alt newsgroup, please
- contact your own News administrator and request that they
- begin carrying that specific group.

Figure 2.66:
This guide to online support groups is available on the Web and is posted to numerous newsgroups and mailing lists.

# Appendices

A: Where Do I Go
   from Here?

B: Internet Service
   Providers

# Where Do I Go from Here?

Now that you know the basics and what is out there on the Internet, you may want to find out more about using the Internet. For example, you may want to learn in more detail about the World Wide Web, Usenet, Gopher, and FTP *and* about the software and tools you can use to make the most of your Internet travels.

You may, for example, want to browse the Web to visit the Virtual Hospital, tunnel through the Gopherspace of the U.S. government's health agencies, or learn to FTP recipes and fitness documents from some of the Internet's computer archives.

If you'd like a basic, plain English tour of the Internet and its uses, *A Guided Tour of the Internet* by Christian Crumlish is for you. It's like having an Internet guru at your side, explaining everything as you go along. Another great book for newbies is *Access the Internet* by David Peal. This book even includes NetCruiser software, which will get you connected via an easy point-and-click interface in no time.

For an introduction to the World Wide Web, turn to *Mosaic Access to the Internet* or to *Surfing the Internet with Netscape*, both by Daniel A. Tauber and Brenda Kienan. Each of these books walks you through getting connected, and they both include the software you need to get started on the Web in a jiffy.

For quick and easy Internet reference, turn to the *Internet Instant Reference* by Paul Hoffman, and for an in-depth overview, try the best-selling *Internet Roadmap* by Bennett Falk. To get familiar with the lingo, you can turn to the compact and concise *Internet Dictionary* by Christian Crumlish.

If you've just got to learn all there is to know about the Internet, the comprehensive, complete *Mastering the Internet* by Glee Harrah Cady and Pat McGregor is for you. And if you want to find out what tools and utilities are available (often on the Internet itself) to maximize the power of your

Internet experience, you'll want to check out *The Internet Tool Kit* by Nancy Cedeño.

All these books have been published by Sybex in 1995 editions.

# Internet Service Providers

If you want to set up an account with an Internet service provider, this is the place for you. This appendix lists providers in the U.S., Canada, Great Britain, Ireland, Australia, and New Zealand.

*The service providers listed here offer full Internet service, including SLIP/PPP accounts, which allow you to use Web browsers such as Mosaic and Netscape.*

The list here is by no means comprehensive. We're concentrating on service providers that offer national or nearly national Internet service in English-speaking countries. You may prefer to go with a service provider that is local to your area—to minimize your phone bill, it is important to find a service provider that offers a local or toll-free phone number for access.

When you inquire into establishing an account with any of the providers listed in this appendix, tell them the type of account you want. For example, you may want a shell account if you know and plan to use Unix commands to get around, or you may want the type of point-and-click access that's offered through Netcom's Net-Cruiser. If you want to run a Web browser such as Mosaic or Netscape, you must have a SLIP or PPP account. Selecting an Internet service provider is a matter of personal preference and local access. Shop around, and if you aren't satisfied at any point, change providers.

## What's Out There

Two very good sources of information about Internet service providers are available on the Internet itself. Peter Kaminski's Public Dialup Internet Access list (PDIAL) is at

ftp://ftp.netcom.com/pub/in/info-deli/public-access/pdial.

Yahoo's Internet Access Providers list is at

http://www.yahoo.com/Business/COrporations/Internet_Access_providers/.

*When you're shopping around for an Internet service provider, the most important questions to ask are: What is the nearest local access number? What are the monthly service charges? Is there a setup (or registration) fee?*

## IN THE U.S.

In this section we list Internet service providers that offer local access phone numbers in most major U.S. cities. These are the big, national companies. Many areas also have smaller regional Internet providers, which may offer better local access if you're not in a big city. You can find out about these smaller companies by looking in computer publications such as *MicroTimes* and *Computer Currents* or by getting on the Internet via one of the big companies and checking out the Peter Kaminski and Yahoo service provider listings.

*Opening an account with any of the providers listed here will get you full access to the World Wide Web and full-fledged e-mail service (allowing you to send and receive e-mail). You'll also get the ability to read and post articles to Usenet newsgroups.*

### Netcom Online Communications Services
Netcom is a national Internet service provider with local access numbers in most major U.S. cities. (As of this writing, Netcom has 100 local access numbers in the U.S.) Netcom's NetCruiser software gives you point-and-click access to the Internet. (Netcom also provides a shell account, but stay away from it if you want to run Netscape.) Starting with NetCruiser version 1.6, it is possible to run Netscape on top of NetCruiser. Especially for beginning users who want a point-and-click interface and easy setup of Netscape, this may be a good choice.

NetCruiser software is available on disk for free but without documentation at many trade shows and bookstores. It is also available with a very good book (*Access the Internet, Second Edition*; David Peal, Sybex, 1995) that shows you how to use the software.

To contact Netcom directly, phone (800) 353-6600.

### Performance Systems International
Performance Systems International (PSI) is a national Internet service provider that offers local access numbers in many U.S. cities *and in Japan*. The folks at PSI are currently

upgrading their modems to 28.8K bps, which will give you faster access to the Internet.

To contact PSI, phone (800) 82P-SI82.

**UUNet/AlterNet** UUNet Technologies and AlterNet offer Internet service throughout the U.S. They run their own national network.

To contact UUnet and AlterNet, phone (800) 488-6383.

**Portal** Portal Communications, Inc., an Internet service provider in the San Francisco Bay Area, lets you get connected either by dialing one of its San Francisco Bay Area phone numbers or via the CompuServe network. (This is not CompuServe Information Services, but rather the network on which CompuServe runs.) The CompuServe network, with more than 400 access phone numbers, is a local call throughout most of the U.S.

To contact Portal, phone (408) 973-9111.

# IN CANADA

Listed here are providers that offer access to Internet service in the areas around large Canadian cities. For information about local access in less-populated regions, get connected and check out the Peter Kaminski and Yahoo lists described earlier in this appendix.

 *Many Internet service providers in the U.S. also offer service in Canada and in border towns near Canada. If you're interested and you're in Canada, you can ask some of the big U.S. service providers whether they have a local number near you.*

**UUNet Canada** UUNet Canada is the Canadian division of the U.S. service provider UUNet/AlterNet, which we described earlier in this appendix. UUNet Canada offers Internet service to large portions of Canada.

To contact UUNet Canada, phone (416) 368-6621.

**Internet Direct** Internet Direct offers access to folks in the Toronto and Vancouver areas.

To contact Internet Direct, phone (604) 691-1600 or fax (604) 691-1605.

## IN GREAT BRITAIN AND IRELAND

The Internet is, after all, international. Here are some service providers located and offering service in Great Britain and Ireland.

**UNet** Located in the northwest part of England, with more locations promised, UNet offers access at speeds up to 28.8K bps along with various Internet tools for your use.

To contact UNet, phone 0925 633 144.

**Easynet** London-based Easynet provides Internet service throughout England via Pipex, along with a host of Internet tools.

To contact Easynet, phone 0171 209 0990.

**Ireland On-Line10** Serving most (if not all) of Ireland, including Belfast, Ireland On-Line offers complete Internet service including ISDN and leased-line connections.

To contact Ireland On-Line, phone 00 353 (0)1 8551740.

## IN AUSTRALIA AND NEW ZEALAND

Down under in Australia and New Zealand the Internet is as happening as it is in the northern hemisphere; many terrific sites are located in Australia especially. Here are a couple of service providers for that part of the world.

**Connect.com.au** In wild and woolly Australia, Internet service (SLIP/PPP) is available from Connect.com.au Pty Ltd.

To contact Connect.com.au, phone 61 3 528 2239.

**Actrix Information Exchange** Actrix Information Exchange offers Internet service (PPP accounts) in the Wellington, New Zealand area.

To contact Actrix, phone 64 4 389 6316.

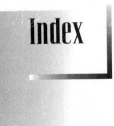

# Index

**Note to the Reader:** Throughout this index **boldfaced** page numbers indicate primary discussions of a topic. *Italicized* page numbers indicate illustrations.

# The Complete Pocket Tour Series from Sybex

*A Pocket Tour of:*

Games on the Internet

Health & Fitness on the Internet

Money on the Internet

Music on the Internet

Sports on the Internet

Travel on the Internet

*with more coming soon to a store near you.*